THE TREATMENT
OF PARKINSONISM
WITH L-DOPA

THE TREATMENT OF PARKINSONISM WITH L-DOPA

John Marks

MTP Medical and Technical Publishing Co. Ltd.

Published by
MTP
MEDICAL AND TECHNICAL
PUBLISHING CO LTD
PO Box 55, St. Leonard's House
St. Leonard Gate
Lancaster, Lancs.

ISBN 978-94-015-7232-3   ISBN 978-94-015-7230-9 (eBook)

DOI 10.1007/978-94-015-7230-9

Contents

CONTENTS

PART 1.   INTRODUCTION   1

PART 2.   THE ORIGINAL DESCRIPTION OF "THE SHAKING   7
           PALSY"
           Paper: James Parkinson, – Extracts from "An
           Essay on the Shaking Palsy" – London 1817

PART 3.   THE FIRST IMPLICATION OF THE MID-BRAIN AND
           SUBSTANTIA NIGRA IN THE PATHOGENESIS OF THE
           DISEASE
           Paper: Trétiakoff C., Contribution à l'Etude de
           l'Anatomie Pathologique du Locus Niger de
           Soemmering avec Quelque Déductions Relative
           à la Pathogenie des Troubles du Tonus Muscul-
           aire et de la Maladie de Parkinsonism. Thesis,
           Paris 1919 (*Translation*)

PART 4.   CHEMISTRY   29
           Paper: Guggenheim M., Dioxyphenylalanin, eine
           neue Aminosäure aus vicia faba *Z. Physiol.
           Chem.*, **88**, 276, 1913 (*Translation*)

PART 5.   THE RECOGNITION OF AN ACTION OF DOPAMINE IN   39
          THE BRAIN
          Paper: Carlsson A., Lindquist M., and Magnus-
          son T., 3, 4, Dihydroxyphenylalanine and 5-
          Hydroxytryptophan as Reserpine Antagonists,
          Nature **180**, 1200, 1957

PART 6.   PATHOPHYSIOLOGICAL FINDINGS IN PARKINSONISM   45
          Paper: Ehringer H., and Hornykiewicz O., Ver-
          teilung von Noradrenalin und Dopamin (3-
          hydroxytyramin) im Gehirn des Menschen und
          ihr Verhalten bei Erkrankungen des Extra-
          pyramidalen Systems, *Klin. Wscher.*, **38**, 1236,
          1960 (*Translation*)

PART 7.   THE INITIAL CLINICAL TRIALS   57
          Paper: Birkmayer W., and Hornykiewicz O.,
          Der L-3,4-Dioxyphenylalanin (=DOPA) Effekt
          bei der Parkinson-Akinese, *Wien klin. Wscher.*,
          73, 787, 1961 (*Translation*)

          Barbeau A., Murphy G. F., and Sourkes T. L.,
          Les Catecholamines dans la Maladie de Parkin-
          son, in Bel-Air Symposium on Monoamines and
          the Central Nervous System, Georg et Cie,
          Geneva 1961 (*Translation*)

PART 8.   TRIALS OF ORAL THERAPY   81
          Paper: Cotzias G. C., Van Woert M. H., and
          Schiffer L. M., Aromatic Amino Acids and
          Modification of Parkinsonism, *New Eng. J. Med.*,
          276, 374, 1967

PART 9.   RELATIONSHIP OF LEVODOPA TO OTHER FORMS OF   99
          THERAPY
          Paper: Hughes R. C., Polgar J. G., Weightman
          D., and Walton J. N., Levodopa in Parkinsonism:
          The Effects of Withdrawal of Anticholinergic
          Drugs, *Brit . med. J.*, **2**, 487, 1971

PART 10.   THE RATIONALE AND EXPERIENCE OF THE CON-   117
            COMITANT ADMINISTRATION OF DECARBOXYLASE
            INHIBITORS AND LEVODOPA
            Paper: Pletscher A., and Bartholini G., Selective
            Rise in Brain Dopamine by Inhibition of Extra
            cerebral Levodopa Decarboxylation, *Clin. Phar-
            macol. Ther.*, **12**, 344, 1970

            Barbeau A., Gillo-Joffrey L., and Mars H.,
            Treatment of Parkinson's Disease with Levodopa
            and Ro4-4602, *Clin. Pharmacol. Ther.*, 1970, **12**,
            353

PART 11.   METABOLIC AND BIOCHEMICAL ACTIONS   143
            Paper: Calne D. B., and Sandler M., L-Dopa and
            Parkinsonism, *Nature*, **226**, 21, 1970

PART 12.   FURTHER PROBLEMS   157

            APPENDIX. CURRENT VIEWS ON THE CLINICAL USE   159
            OF LEVODOPA

Part 1

Introduction

John Marks

There are two separate ways by which therapeutic advances can occur—serendipity (chance observation) or as a direct result of clinical studies arising from the application of the results of basic research. The use of levodopa in the treatment of Parkinsonism is a prime example of the latter. Although disorders broadly described as "shaking palsy" had been described over the centuries since the time of Galen, the classic description of the disease is that published by James Parkinson in 1817, under the title "Paralysis Agitans". Charcot, some forty years later, suggested that the disease should bear the eponym "Parkinson's Disease", the name by which it has since been known. Strictly speaking Parkinsonism is a more appropriate term, for it is a chronic neurological syndrome which may result from many causes and is characterised by rigidity, hypokinesia and tremor.

Parkinsonism is a relatively common disorder with an estimated prevalence of between 1.0 and 1.5 per 1000 in developed communities. Indeed it may afflict up to perhaps 1 per cent of those over fifty years of age, although the latter figure has been disputed. In most sufferers, at the present time, the initial symptoms and signs do not develop until the fifth or sixth decade. In the 1930s Parkinsonism was usually a sequel of the pandemic viral infection encephalitis lethargica of the late twenties, but happily is now rare. The majority of current cases are classified as idiopathic, although perhaps with a genetic background, though it is possible that they still represent late sequelae from the encephalitis pandemic. A suggestion has been made that atherosclerotic lesions may be involved, and in this age group co-incidental association would not be surprising. Iatrogenic Parkinsonism is now all too

1

common, associated with the administration inter alia *of rauwolfia alkaloids and related substances (e.g. reserpine and tetrabenazine); phenothiazine tranquillisers (e.g. chlorpromazine, perphenazine); butyrophenones (e.g. haloperidol) and occasionally methyldopa. Among rare causes of the disorder are traumatic encephalopathy; various toxins (e.g. manganese, carbon monoxide) tumours of the basal ganglia, or other tumours leading to mid brain compression.*

The main clinical features are tremor which is often reduced during voluntary movement; rigidity usually with a flexed posture; slowness of initiation of movement; dysarthria and dysphagia; festinant gait; hypokinesia with the mask-like facies; ocular manifestations such as infrequent blinking, oculogyric crises; alimentary disorders, particularly drooling saliva and constipation; and in many patients seborrhoea. The majority of these clinical manifestations are described in the original account of the disorder by James Parkinson (see Part 2).

Parkinsonism is the result of abnormal activity within the substantia nigra and basal ganglia components of the extrapyramidal system. This system utilises input information from the muscle spindles and polysynaptic feedback loops to produce smooth and integrated movements mainly by modulating corticospinal activity. The exact interrelations of the basal ganglia nuclei are far from clear but as with many other parts of the central nervous system, a balance between excitatory and inhibitory loops is probably important. The effects of these excitatory and inhibitory feedback loops are in their turn transmitted to the anterior horn cells and thence via the "final common path" to the muscles. The existing evidence suggests that some of these influences (mainly those concerned with rigidity) are relayed via the nucleus giganto cellularis, a nucleus of the reticular formation, and that these then affect the α motor neuron directly. On the other hand, the main path for tremor control appears to be via the thalamus, the motor cortex, pyramidal tract and the γ efferent system. The excitatory and inhibitory loops in the basal ganglia in their turn depend upon different synaptic transmitters and dopamine, acetylcholine, serotonin and perhaps histamine and noradrenaline may be involved. One current hypothesis suggests that one vital balance is between an inhibitory dopaminergic nigrostriatal pathway and a neighbouring excitatory cholinergic pathway which also acts on the corpus striatum. The first step in the understanding of Parkinsonism was the finding of degenerate lesions in the substantia nigra, with depigmentation, cell vacuolation and intraneural inclusion bodies known as Lewy bodies. This discovery occurred at the beginning of this century (see Part 3).

Although the pathological anatomy was largely understood by the 1920s, it

2

was a further thirty years before the next advance was made. As with many recent advances in current neurophysiology it stemmed from the studies in psychopharmacology. It had been shown in animals (see Part 5) that the extrapyramidal manifestations of reserpine were due to a deficiency in brain dopamine. Dopamine will not cross the blood-brain barrier whereas the precursor amino acid levodopa will (see Part 4) and the administration of this compound corrected the deficiency and alleviated the symptoms.

Details of the metabolic pathways for levodopa and the chemical formulae of the substances involved are given in Part 11. They are summarised in Figure 1 which shows that several known physiologically active compounds are formed together with others that may have pharmacological activity in the nervous system or elsewhere in the body.

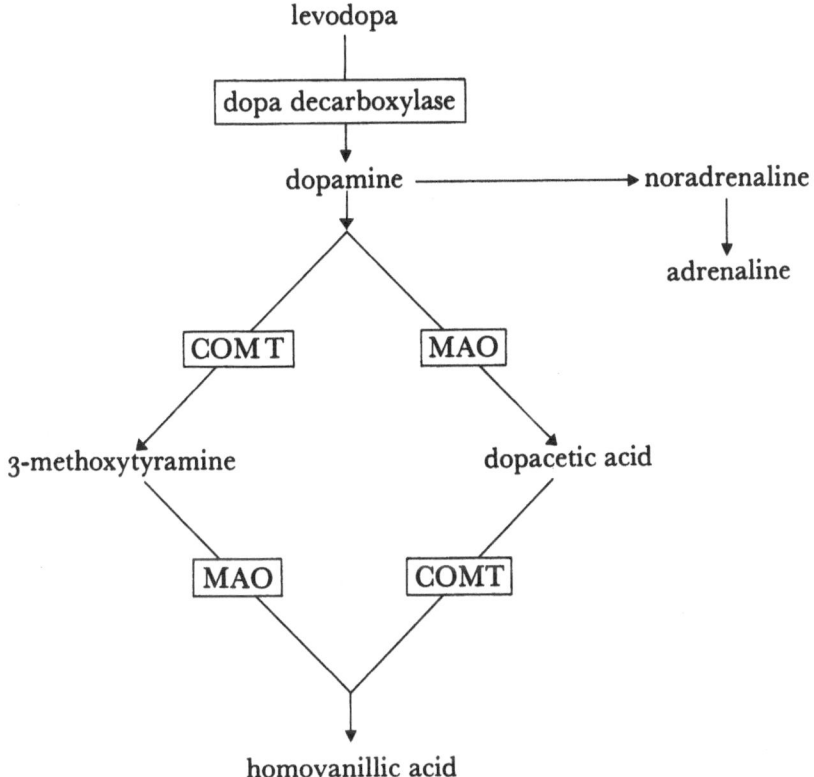

Fig. 1. — Summary of metabolic paths of levodopa. The enzymes are shown in boxes. COMT = catechclortho methyl transferase; MAO = monoamine oxidase.

The Treatment of Parkinsonism with L-Dopa

The practical human importance of this observation might not have emerged without the demonstration in 1960 by Ehringer and Hornykiewicz (see Part 6) that the normally high concentration of dopamine in the human corpus striatum was markedly reduced in patients with Parkinsonism. This led quite logically to the clinical studies of levodopa both in Vienna and Montreal (Part 7) and the subsequent confirmatory trials of high and maintained oral doses of levodopa (Part 8).

Thus in 1967 the merits and problems of large oral doses of levodopa were established. It was found that good relief can be expected to occur in some 60 per cent of patients. The last five years have seen extensive trials to determine the optimum regimen with other agents (e.g. anticholinergics, amantadine —see Part 9) and with peripheral decarboxylase inhibitors (to potentiate the central nervous system effects—see Part 10).

The substances which provoke Parkinsonism or can influence its course act by different mechanisms. These are not yet totally understood but the current ideas of the possible mechanisms are shown in Figure 2. On this basis it might be supposed that with such a logical approach the problems of treatment of Parkinsonism with levodopa are solved. Unfortunately this is not so. It is still far from clear whether the increase of brain dopamine is the prime cause of the response to levodopa and since 90 per cent of the patients experience side-effects to a greater or lesser degree levodopa cannot be regarded as the ideal therapeutic agent (Part 8, 11 and 12), but it is still regarded as the most effective treatment which is currently available.

The era in which levodopa as the drug of choice for Parkinsonism may well be short and may be superseded by other drug combinations, perhaps including levodopa, or by better drugs. Nevertheless the history of the discovery and development of levodopa therapy is an excellent demonstration of basic research leading to a logical treatment.

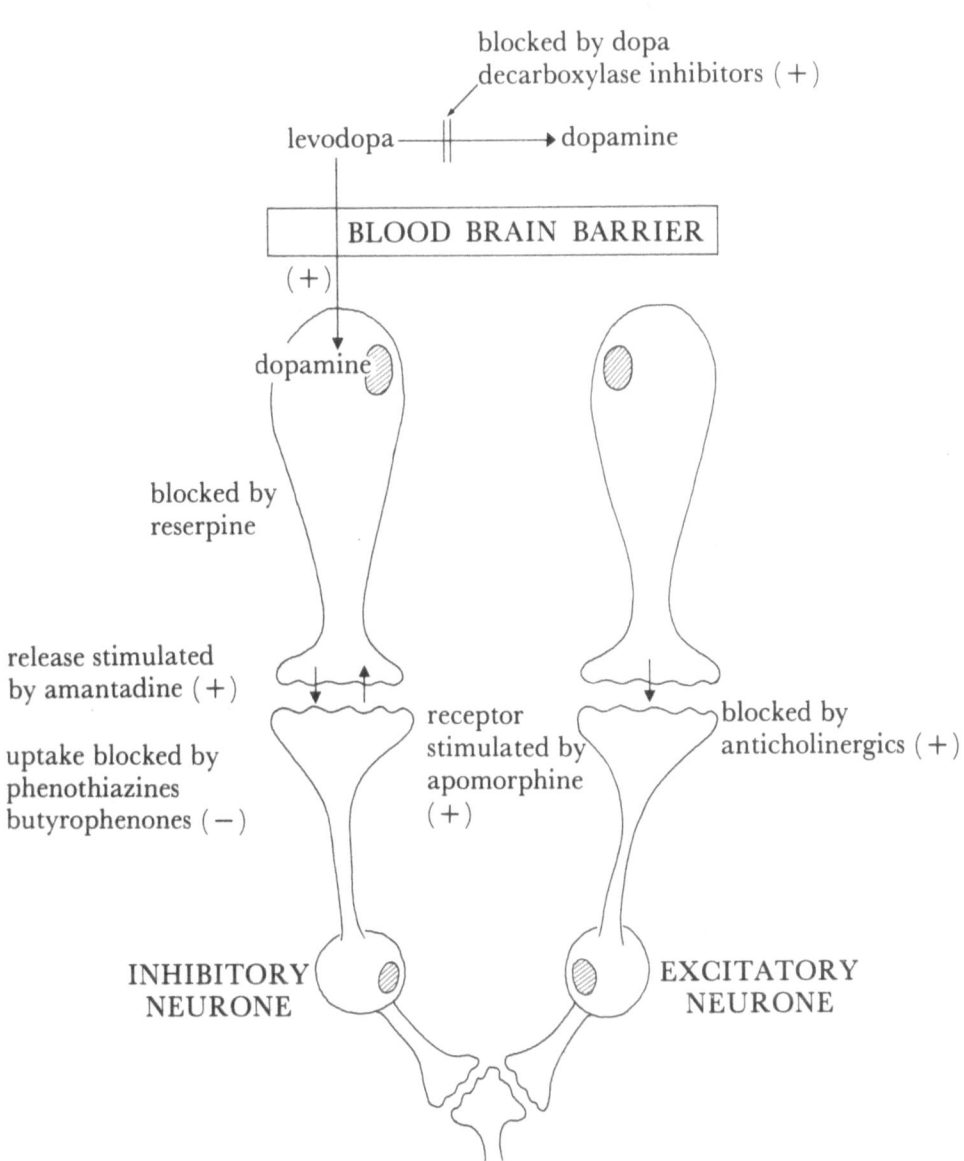

Fig. 2. — Representation of mechanisms by which therapeutic substances may affect Parkinsonism. (+) signifies improvement, (−) signifies deterioration.

Part 2

The Original Description of "The Shaking Palsy"

Although the book is primarily concerned with the development of ideas on the therapy of "paralysis agitans" with levodopa it seems to be appropriate to start with the brilliant description by James Parkinson of the disease that now bears his name.

James Parkinson (1755–1824) was born in Shoreditch, son of a local apothecary and surgeon, and spent his whole medical life as a general practitioner there. At that period Shoreditch was a small but prosperous market town near London surrounded by meadows and streams. Little is known about Parkinson's medical practice, but in addition to his prolific writing on many medical topics which show him to have been a modest, skilful and conscientious practitioner, he was also a noted geologist and an ardent political reformer.

His most famous publication "An Essay on the Shaking Palsy" was published when he was sixty two years old. It described his observations on six patients. He recorded in fact most of the features of the condition in one of the classic papers of medical history. The reader is moreover directed to the caution and self-deprecation that are features of the preface. The synonyms "shaking palsy" and "paralysis agitans" had, as he points out, been used by many previous medical writers as far back as Galen for a mixed group of diseases and it was Parkinson who first recognised that certain features were common to one disorder, or strictly speaking to a closely related group of disorders. That is, Parkinsonism is strictly a syndrome.

He noted the slow but relentless progress of the disease and drew specific attention to the increasing tremor at rest, which he noted sometimes subsided during voluntary movement; the festinant gait; the flexed posture; the dysarthria and dysphagia; the insomnia; the severe constipation. The only cardinal features which he did not mention and which would now be regarded as essential for a diagnosis of Parkinsonism were the muscular rigidity with slowness of initiation of movement and the facial immobility.

It was Charcot some forty years later who regarded the term "paralysis agitans" as a misnomer when muscular strength was well preserved and tremor might be lacking and who proposed that the disorder should be known as Parkinson's Disease.

James Parkinson had no idea of the pathology of this disorder and regarded the cause as damage of the cervical spinal cord and the medulla with no disorder of the cerebral hemispheres as exemplified by the preservation of intellectual function. He had no real advice to give on therapy for the disease, but two specific sentences appear worthy of direct quotation for they represent not only the ideal general approach to medical research, but point the way to the current therapy in the disorder that now carries his name.

"Until we are better informed respecting the nature of this disease, the employment of internal medicines is scarcely warrantable; unless analogy should point out some remedy the trial of which rational hope might authorise", and:

"Before concluding these pages, it may be proper to observe once more, that an important object proposed to be obtained by them is the leading of the attention of those who humanely employ anatomical examination in detecting the causes and nature of diseases, particularly to this malady".

The original essay is almost 11000 words long and a full reprint would place too great a stress on this part of a book which is primarily concerned with the developments of therapy. An annotated abridged version is therefore given.

Editor's Note.

The use of *d, l*-dopa and D, L-Dopa throughout this book has been left unchanged in the original papers, although D, L is the accepted notation today.

Reprinted from An Essay on the Shaking Palsy, by James Parkinson, (Sherwood, Neely and Jones: London 1817)

AN ESSAY ON THE SHAKING PALSY

JAMES PARKINSON
MEMBER OF THE ROYAL COLLEGE OF SURGEONS

PREFACE

The advantages which have been derived from the caution with which hypothetical statements are admitted, are in no instance more obvious than in those sciences which more particularly belong to the healing art. It therefore is necessary, that some conciliatory explanation should be offered for the present publication: in which, it is acknowledged, that mere conjecture takes the place of experiment; and, that analogy is the substitute for anatomical examination, the only sure foundation for pathological knowledge.

When, however, the nature of the subject, and the circumstances under which it has been here taken up, are considered, it is hoped that the offering of the following pages to the attention of the medical public, will not be severely censured. The disease, respecting which the present inquiry is made, is of a nature highly afflictive. Notwithstanding which, it has not yet obtained a place in the classification of nosologists; some have regarded its characteristic symptoms as distinct and different diseases, and others have given its name to diseases differing essentially from it; whilst the unhappy sufferer has considered it as an evil, from the domination of which he had no prospect of escape.

The disease is of long duration: to connect, therefore, the symptoms which occur in its later stages with those which mark its commencement, requires a continuance of observation of the same

9

case, or at least a correct history of its symptoms, even for several years. Of both these advantages the writer has had the opportunities of availing himself; and has hence been led particularly to observe several other cases in which the disease existed in different stages of its progress. By these repeated observations, he hoped that he had been led to a probable conjecture as to the nature of the malady, and that analogy had suggested such means as might be productive of relief, and perhaps even of cure, if employed before the disease had been too long established. He therefore considered it to be a duty to submit his opinions to the examination of others, even in their present state of immaturity and imperfection.

CHAPTER I

DEFINITION — HISTORY — ILLUSTRATIVE CASES

SHAKING PALSY (*Paralysis Agitans*)

Involuntary tremulous motion, with lessened muscular power, in parts not in action and even when supported; with a propensity to bend the trunk forwards, and to pass from a walking to a running pace: the senses and intellects being uninjured.

The term Shaking Palsy has been vaguely employed by medical writers in general. By some it has been used to designate ordinary cases of Palsy, in which some slight tremblings have occurred; whilst by others it has been applied to certain anomalous affections, not belonging to Palsy.

The shaking of the limbs belonging to this disease was particularly noticed, as will be seen when treating of the symptoms, by Galen, who marked its peculiar character by an appropriate term. The same symptom was accurately treated of by Sylvius de la Boe. Juncker also seems to have referred to this symptom: having divided tremor into active and passive. . . .

. . . Tremor can indeed only be considered as a symptom, although several species of it must be admitted. In the present instance, the agitation produced by the peculiar species of tremor, which here occurs, is chosen to furnish the epithet by which this species of Palsy, may be distinguished.

"The Shaking Palsy"

HISTORY

So slight and nearly imperceptible are the first inroads of this malady, and so extremely slow is its progress, that it rarely happens, that the patient can form any recollection of the precise period of its commencement. The first symptoms perceived are, a slight sense of weakness, with a proneness to trembling in some particular part; sometimes in the head, but most commonly in one of the hands and arms. These symptoms gradually increase in the part first affected; and at an uncertain period, but seldom in less than twelve months or more, the morbid influence is felt in some other part. Thus assuming one of the hands and arms to be first attacked, the other, at this period becomes similarly affected. After a few more months the patient is found to be less strict than usual in preserving an upright posture: this being most observable whilst walking, but sometimes whilst sitting or standing. Sometime after the appearance of this symptom, and during its slow increase, one of the legs is discovered slightly to tremble, and is also found to suffer fatigue sooner than the leg of the other side: and in a few months this limb becomes agitated by similar tremblings, and suffers a similar loss of power. . . .

Hitherto the patient will have experienced but little inconvenience . . . [*except*] . . . whilst writing or employing himself in any nicer kind of manipulation. But as the disease proceeds, similar employments are accomplished with considerable difficulty, the hand failing to answer with exactness to the dictates of the will. Walking . . . becomes a task which cannot be performed without considerable attention. The legs are not raised to that height, or with that promptitude which the will directs, so that the utmost care is necessary to prevent frequent falls.

At this period the patient experiences much inconvenience, which unhappily is found daily to increase. . . .

. . . Writing can now be hardly at all accomplished; and reading, from the tremulous motion, is accomplished with some difficulty. Whilst at meals the fork not being duly directed frequently fails to raise the morsel from the plate: which, when seized, is with much difficulty conveyed to the mouth. At this period the patient seldom experiences a suspension of the agitation of his limbs. Commencing, for instance in one arm, the wearisome agitation is borne until beyond sufferance, when by suddenly changing the posture it is for a time stopped in that limb, to commence, generally in less than a minute in one of the legs, or in the arm of the other side.

Harassed by this tormenting round, the patient has recourse to walking, a mode of exercise to which the sufferers from this malady are in general partial; owing to their attention being thereby somewhat diverted from their unpleasant feelings, by the care and exertion required to ensure its safe performance.

But as this malady proceeds, even this temporary mitigation of suffering from the agitation of the limbs is denied. The propensity to lean forward becomes invincible, and the patient is thereby forced to step on the toes and fore part of the feet, whilst the upper part of the body is thrown so far forward as to render it difficult to avoid falling on the face. In some cases, when this state of the malady is attained, the patient can no longer exercise himself by walking in his usual manner, but is thrown on the toes and forepart of the feet; being, at the same time, irresistibly impelled to take much quicker and shorter steps, and thereby to adopt unwillingly a running pace. . . .

In this stage, the sleep becomes much disturbed. The tremulous motion of the limbs occur during sleep, and augment until they awaken the patient, and frequently with much agitation and alarm. The power of conveying the food to the mouth is at length so much impeded that he is obliged to consent to be fed by others. The bowels, which had been all along torpid, now, in most cases, demand stimulating medicines of very considerable power: the expulsion of the faeces from the rectum sometimes requiring mechanical aid. As the disease proceeds towards its last stage, the trunk is almost permanently bowed, the muscular power is more decidedly diminished, and the tremulous agitation becomes violent. The patient walks now with great difficulty, and unable any longer to support himself with his stick, he dares not venture on this exercise, unless assisted by an attendant, who walking backwards before him, prevents his falling forwards, by the pressure of his hands against the fore part of his shoulder and he is not only no longer able to feed himself, but when the food is conveyed to the mouth, so much are the actions of the muscles of the tongue, pharynx, &c. impeded by impaired action and perpetual agitation, that the food is with difficulty retained in the mouth until masticated; and then as difficultly swallowed. Now also, from the same cause, another very unpleasant circumstance occurs: the saliva fails of being directed to the back part of the fauces, and hence is continually draining from the mouth, mixed with the particles of food, which he is no longer able to clear from the inside of the mouth.

As the debility increases and the influence of the will over the muscle fades away, the tremulous agitation becomes more vehement. It now seldom leaves him for a moment; but even when exhausted nature seizes a small portion of sleep, the motion becomes so violent as not only to shake the bed-hangings, but even the floor and sashes of the room. The chin is now almost immoveably bent down upon the sternum. The slops with which he is attempted to be fed, with the saliva, are continually trickling from the mouth. The power of articulation is lost. The urine and faeces are passed involuntarily; and at the last, constant sleepiness, with slight delirium, and other marks of extreme exhaustion, announce the wished-for release.

Doctor Parkinson then describes the six cases he has seen on which his account of the disorder is based, viz: —

Case 1   A gardener of over 50 years of age of whom only minimal details are given.

Case 2   An attendant at a magistrate's office who at 62 "was casually met with in the street" ... "he had suffered from the disorder about eight or ten years" *and was then in a moderately advanced state of disorder.*

Case 3   The man of about 65 years of age "was also noticed casually in the street". *He had been a sailor who had been confined in a Spanish prison.* "The disorder had here continued so long and made such a progress as to afford little or no prospect of relief".

Case 4   This was a "gentleman of about 55 years who had first experienced the trembling of the arms about five years before." *Doctor Parkinson treated him for a chest abscess and the patient then moved* "to a distant part of the country" *preventing prolonged observation.*

Case 5   This was a gentleman, accompanied by his attendant, who was seen at a distance in the street but demonstrated the festinant gait to a marked degree.

Case 6   This gentleman at 72 is described in the greatest detail. He had suffered from the disorder for "about 11 or 12, or perhaps more years" *and this was now in a rather advanced state.*

13

CHAPTER II

PATHOGNOMONIC SYMPTOMS EXAMINED

It has been seen in the preceding history of the disease, and in the accompanying cases, that certain affections, the tremulous agitations, and the almost invincible propensity to run, when wishing only to walk, each of which has been considered by nosologists as distinct diseases, appear to be pathognomonic symptoms of this malady.

The author then considers specific symptoms in detail—the tremor, the forward bend in the trunk and the festinant gait. He describes what previous writers have said about them, particularly Juncker, Sylvius de la Böe, Gaubius and Sauvage.
On the tremor Doctor Parkinson writes as follows:

. . . . It is also necessary to bear in mind, that this affection is distinguishable from tremor, by the agitation, in the former, occurring whilst the affected part is supported and unemployed, and being even checked by the adoption of voluntary motion; whilst in the latter, the tremor is induced immediately on bringing the parts into action. Thus an artist, afflicted with the malady here treated of, whilst his hand and arm is palpitating strongly, will seize his pencil, and the motions will be suspended, allowing him to use it for a short period; but in tremor, if the hand be quite free from the affection should the pen or pencil be taken up, the trembling immediately commences.

CHAPTER III

SHAKING PALSY DISTINGUISHED FROM OTHER DISEASES WITH WHICH IT MAY BE CONFOUNDED

Treating of a disease resulting from an assemblage of symptoms, some of which do not appear to have yet engaged the general notice of the profession, particular care is required whilst endeavouring to mark its diagnostic characters.

Doctor Parkinson then describes other disorders which might be termed "Shaking Palsy" but which must be distinguished from the syndrome he describes. He concludes as follows:

14

Unless attention is paid to one circumstance, this disease will be confounded with those species of passive tremblings to which the term Shaking Palsies has frequently been applied. These are, *tremor temulentus*, the trembling consequent to indulgence in the drinking of spirituous liquors; that which proceeds from the immoderate employment of tea and coffee: that which appears to be dependent on advanced age; and all those tremblings which proceed from the various circumstances which induce a diminution of power in the nervous system. But by attending to that circumstance alone, which has been already noted as characteristic of mere tremor, the distinction will readily be made. If the trembling limb be supported, and none of its muscles be called into action, the trembling will cease. In the real Shaking Palsy the reverse of this takes place, the agitation continues in full force whilst the limb is at rest and unemployed: and even is sometimes diminished by calling the muscles into employment.

CHAPTER IV

PROXIMATE CAUSE—REMOTE CAUSES—ILLUSTRATIVE CASES

Before making the attempt to point out the nature and cause of this disease, it is necessary to plead, that it is made under very unfavourable circumstances. Unaided by previous inquiries immediately directed to this disease, and not having had the advantage, in a single case, of that light which anatomical examination yields, opinions and not facts can only be offered. Conjecture founded on analogy, and an attentive consideration of the peculiar symptoms of the disease, have been the only guides that could be obtained for this research, the result of which is, as it ought to be, offered with hesitation.

SUPPOSED PROXIMATE CAUSE

A diseased state of the *medulla spinalis*, in that part which is contained in the canal, formed by the superior cervical vertebrae, and extending, as the disease proceeds, to the *medulla oblongata*.

Uncertainty existing as the nature of the proximate cause of this disease, its remote causes must necessarily be referred to with indecision. Assuming however the state just mentioned as the proximate cause, it may be concluded that this may be the result of injuries of the medulla itself, or of the theca helping to form the canal in which it is enclosed.

Doctor Parkinson then reviews both the clinical manifestations and autopsy findings of certain other patients with paralysis and tremor as symptoms. In some of these abnormalities were present in the medulla. Though he recognised that these cases did not represent examples of the syndrome that he had described, he felt that medullary disorders might be the main cause of paralysis agitans. Nevertheless he stated:

It must be too obvious that the evidence adduced as to the nature of the proximate and occasional causes of this disease, is by no means conclusive.

CHAPTER V

CONSIDERATIONS RESPECTING THE MEANS OF CURE

The inquiries made in the preceding pages yield, it is to be much regretted, but little more than evidence of inference: nothing direct and satisfactory has been obtained. All that has been ventured to assume here, has been that the disease depends on a disordered state of that part of the medulla which is contained in the cervical vertebrae. But of what nature that morbid change is; and whether originating in the medulla itself, in its membranes, or in the containing theca, is, at present, the subject of doubt and conjecture. But although, at present, uninformed as to the precise nature of the disease, still it ought not to be considered as one against which there exists no countervailing remedy.

On the contrary, there appears to be sufficient reason for hoping that some remedial process may ere long be discovered, by which, at least, the progress of the disease may be stopped. It seldom happens that the agitation extends beyond the arms within the first two years; which period, therefore, if we were disposed to divide the disease into stages, might be said to comprise the first stage. In this period, it is very probable, that remedial means might be employed with success; and even, if unfortunately deferred to a later period, they might then arrest the farthest progress of the disease, although the removing of the effects already produced, might be hardly to be expected. . . .

Doctor Parkinson reviewed the possible remedies that might be used including blood letting from the neck, the application of vesicants, mercury and the administration of purgatives. Nevertheless he cautiously commented:

Until we are better informed respecting the nature of this disease, the employment of internal medicines is scarcely warrantable; unless analogy should point out some remedy the trial of which rational hope might authorize.

The two concluding paragraphs of his Essay are particularly characteristic of Doctor James Parkinson, the cautious, scientific observer.

Before concluding these pages, it may be proper to observe once more, that an important object proposed to be obtained by them is, the leading of the attention of those who humanely employ anatomical examination in detecting the causes and nature of diseases, particularly to this malady. By their benevolent labours its real nature may be ascertained, and appropriate modes of relief, or even of cure, pointed out.

To such researches the healing art is already much indebted for the enlargement of its powers of lessening the evils of suffering humanity. Little is the public aware of the obligations it owes to those who, led by professional ardour, and the dictates of duty, have devoted themselves to these pursuits under circumstances. . . .

Every person of consideration and feeling, may judge of the advantages yielded by the philanthropic exertions of a HOWARD; but how few can estimate the benefits bestowed on mankind, by the labours of a MORGAGNI, HUNTER, or BAILLIE.

Part 3

The First Implications of the Midbrain and Substantia Nigra in the Pathogenesis of the Disease

In his original description James Parkinson considered that the prime cause of paralysis agitans was damage of the cervical spinal cord and the medulla. Although Charcot in the nineteenth century had done much to differentiate various conditions characterised by tremor he had offered no alternative ideas about their pathology. This famous nineteenth century French neurologist and neuro-anatomist believed that paralysis agitans was a neurosis and attempted to cure it with psychotherapy.

The first implication of the midbrain is usually ascribed to Blocq and Marinesco (Blocq P, and Marinesco G., Compte Rendus de la Societe de Biologie *Paris* **5**, *105, 1893) but this must be regarded as somewhat tenuous for it was based on one case with unilateral Parkinsonism who at necropsy showed a circumscribed lesion of the contralateral substantia nigra area. Shortly after this it was suggested that idopathic Parkinsonism might be due to nigral lesions (Brissaud E.,* Leçons sur les Maladies Nerveuses, *Paris, Masson, 1895) but the classic description was published in 1919.*

In that year Trétiakoff (Trétiakoff C., Contribution à L'Etude de l'Anatomie Pathologique du Locus Niger de Sommering avec Quelques Déductions Relative à Pathogenie des Troubles du Tonus Musculaire et de la Maladie de Parkinsonism, *Paris Thesis 1919) studied the brains of nine patients with Parkinsonism as part of a more general study of brain histopathology. He found degeneration to, and reduction in the number of pigmented cells of the substantia nigra, together with cytoplasmic inclusions in some of the cells. The whole of this thesis is very extensive and only a small portion is directly concerned with the pathology of Parkinsonism. A translation of this section is given.*

In fact the understanding of the pathological anatomy of this syndrome has relied almost entirely on French workers for most of the remaining features were described by Foix and Nicolesco (Foix C., and Nicolesco J., Anatomie cerebrale: les Noyaux gris Centraux et la Region Misencephalo-sous-optique. *Paris, Masson, 1925).*

Translated from C. Trétiakoff (Thesis for doctorate in Medicine), Faculté de Médicine de Paris, 1919

CONTRIBUTION TO THE STUDY OF THE PATHOLOGICAL ANATOMY OF THE LOCUS NIGER OF SOEMMERING WITH SOME DEDUCTIONS RELATING TO THE PATHOGENESIS OF DISORDERS OF MUSCULAR TONE AND OF PARKINSON'S DISEASE

C. TRÉTIAKOFF

FACULTÉ DE MEDICINE DE PARIS

Lesions of the Locus Niger (= Substantia nigra) in Parkinson's Disease

1. *History of the study of the pathogenesis of Parkinson's Disease*

Parkinson (1817) and other authors, who were among the first (Skoda, Luys) to study the pathogenesis of paralysis agitans, were inclined to attribute it to lesions of the central nervous system. Then, following numerous anatomo-clinical investigations, the subject became more complicated. The hypotheses proliferated. For a long time, many authors considered paralysis agitans as a neurosis (e.g. Charcot, Gowers, Jaccoud, Eichlost, Strumpell, Grasset, Rouzier, De Grazia, Hirt, Leroux). Other authors mentioned greatly varying lesions as regards both characteristics and localisation, which were considered to play a more or less important part in the pathogenesis of this disease. Such lesions were found in:

The peripheral nerves and muscles (Leyden, Borgherini, Hayaschi, Joffroy, Letscher, Redlich, Ratner, Sass, Blocq, Gauthier, Catola, Idelson, Camp, Schiefferdecher).

The glands of internal secretion, especially the parathyroids (Berkeley, Roussy and Clunet).

The spinal cord (Demange, Dubief, Dana, Ballet, Faure, Redlich, Wallenberg, Burzio, Ratner, Caterina, Gordinier, Ketscher).

The spinal ganglia (Burzio, Borgherini).

The medulla (Borgherini, Dana).

The pons (Alquier).
The cerebellum (Naka, Moriyasu).
The cerebral cortex (Souques, Philipp, Wallenberg, Naka, Dana).

On careful analysis, none of these lesions seemed either constant or pathognomonic of paralysis agitans and the majority of them can be considered as being generally due to the advanced age of the patients. However, of greater importance was the localisation of pathogenic lesions at the level of the basic grey ganglia of the peduncular subthalamic area. In effect, the circumscribed lesions (tumours, softening) seem to be in a relation of cause and effect with a unilateral or even monoplegic "Parkinsonian syndrome" and were always situated in the areas referred to (e.g. Mendel, Bouchut, Becehet, Blocq and Marinesco, Dutil, Leyden, Boucher).

It was then that Brissaud, based on the cases of Blocq and Marinesco and on certain theoretical considerations, stated the hypothesis that "a lesion of the Locus Niger (= substantia nigra) could well be the anatomical substratum of Parkinson's disease". In addition, he called attention to the existence of muscular tone disorders in paralysis agitans and he considered that the Parkinsonian rigidity result from the exaggeration of the muscular tone. However at present the majority of authors admit that Parkinson's disease is caused by one or several lesions of the nerve centres. Disagreement arises when it is a question of localising these lesions. The following are the principal localisations:

Substantia Nigra (Brissaud)
Red nucleus (Maillard)
Optic bed (Auton, Nothnagel)
Lenticular nucleus, ganglion of the peduncular ansa, nucleus of the vagus (Lewy), globus pallidus (Hunt)
The white fascia which traverse the subthalamic region:
lenticular ansa with its nucleus, the fields of Forel, the striate fibres and the thalamic pallidus (Ielgersma).

2. *Results of our own investigations*

Our own investigations regarding the histopathology of the substantia nigra and its relationship with the muscular tone disorders demonstrated that there is a cause and effect relationship between the destructive lesions of substantia nigra and the appearance of the principal symptoms of Parkinson's disease, i.e. rigidity and tremor. The reasons suggesting this conclusion are the following:

The Facts

1. In nine cases of paralysis agitans studied by us, the lesions of the substantia nigra appeared to be absolutely constant.
2. In the case of unilateral form of paralysis agitans, the substantia nigra was affected only on the opposite side.
3. In the cases of the unilateral form of paralysis agitans, published by Blocq and Marinesco, Bechet, and Mendel, the substantia nigra showed changes on the opposite side.
4. We constantly observed lesions of the substantia nigra in diseases such as: catatonic form of paralysis agitans; lethargic encephalitis with catatonia; senile tremor and intentional tremor; and in these different diseases the principal Parkinsonian phenomena, rigidity and tremor, are present in a more isolated fashion.
5. In addition to Parkinson's disease, we observed lesions of the substantia nigra following two conditions:

    a) Coinciding with phenomena in which muscular tone disorders play a principal part, such as: acute chorea, multiple sclerosis, torticollis (in the latter the lesions of the substantia nigra are found on the side opposed to the affected muscle group).

    b) Coinciding with severe motor disorders such as those in hemiplegia with contracture, chronic poliomyelitis or transverse myelitis. In these circumstances it is not surprising that no milder or more complex motor disorders are observed. This is also so in cases of haemorrhage and voluminous tumours invading a large part of the brain stem, with a grave general condition and rapid development.

6. We found no contradictory case among our own material or in the medical literature.

In the domain of hypotheses we arrived at the same conclusions by considering the muscular tone disorders as the principal phenomena in paralysis agitans, phenomena ruled by mesencephalic centres, among them certainly the substantia nigra. The latter could be the sympathetic regulatory centre of tonus. We do not pretend to have observed isolated lesions of the substantia nigra in an otherwise completely normal environment of nerve centres. On the contrary, in our patients because of advanced age there exist diffuse and multiple arteriosclerotic lesions. We have already stated that a lesion affecting only the substantia nigra has not been observed to exist.

The fact on which we based our opinion is the perfect and constant coincidence of lesions of the substantia nigra with disorders of tone and the absence of contradictory cases in which the substantia nigra is affected without any accompanying disorders of tone.

3. *Discussion*

On comparing our concepts regarding Parkinson's disease with the concepts of the various authors, we should mention in the first place that our investigation constitutes a simple confirmation of the brilliant hypothesis of Brissaud: "a lesion of the substantia nigra could well be the anatomical substratum of Parkinson's disease".

Among the opinions that are in disagreement with our own, that of Ielgersma becomes less so when one considers that the lenticular ansa as well as its centre of origin are but little known and that we ignore completely the type of fibres of its posterior extremity which are lost between the red nucleus and the substantia nigra.

Let us recall Maillard's hesitation in choosing between the red nucleus and the substantia nigra as the pathogenic centre of paralysis agitans. The author considers its localisation is probable but is not certain. Furthermore, this opinion, being based solely on theoretical reflections, was invalidated by histopathological investigations carried out by Ielgersma and then by Lewy who found that the red nucleus is normal in paralysis agitans. We have examined the red nucleus in all our cases, both by transversal cuts and longitudinal sections and in no case did we observe obvious lesions in this region.

Concerning the opinion of Ramsay Hunt and Lewy, who localise the pathogenic lesions in the lenticular nucleus, based (among other reasons) on the existence of Parkinsonian tremor in Wilson's disease. we can oppose this by emphasising that the same tremor exists in Benedict's syndrome.

A lesion situated outside the cerebral peduncles affecting the efferent fibres of the substantia nigra, the paths and endings of which are completely unknown, could perhaps determine more or less typical Parkinsonian phenomena. However, we agree with the opinion of R. Hunt as regards the very interesting hypothesis of Mirto. This author considers the substantia nigra is a cellular group detached from the globus pallidus during the course of phylogenetic development.

We are unable to define the nature of the degenerative lesions of the nerve cells of the substantia nigra which we observed in Parkinson's disease. The other authors who described lesions at the level of the brain stem in Parkinson's disease usually consider these lesions due to cerebral arteriosclerosis (Alzheimer and his school). In three of our cases: arteriosclerosis is indisputable. In contrast in two cases vascular lesions are absent or insignificant and it is impossible to attribute to them the degenerative lesions. Nor were there any traces of inflammatory conditions.

In conclusion, it seems to us impossible to state a definite opinion regarding the nature of these degenerative lesions of the substantia nigra.

Conclusions

A) *Anatomical deductions*

Of 54 causes of disease of the nervous system which we examined, in 29 cases there were changes of the substantia nigra of Soemmering.
The changes occurred in the following disorders:

a) *Inflammatory lesions:*
    Sydenham's chorea, encephalitis lethargica, generalised paralysis, diffuse tuberculoma, subacute poliomyelitis, multiple sclerosis.
b) *Arteriosclerotic:*
    senile tremor, certain cases of paralysis agitans.
c) *Degenerative lesions of undetermined nature:*
    e.g. Parkinson's disease, torticollis, lateral amyotrophic sclerosis, transverse myelitis.

These disorders produce the following changes in the cells of the substantia nigra:

1. Reduction of black pigment (=substantia nigra);
2. Swelling of the cell body with eccentric nucleus;
3. Acute homogeneous degeneration;

25

4. Hypertrophy and fragmentation of the intracellular neuro-fibrils;
5. Grumous degeneration;
6. Appearance of "Lewy bodies";
7. Appearance of binuclear cells.

Neither among our material nor in the medical literature did we find cases in which the lesions were absolutely localised in the substantia nigra. Whatever the morbid process may be, one observes changes in the immediate or more or less removed areas of the substantia nigra.

B) *Physiological deductions*

The lesions of the substantia nigra are always accompanied by motor disorders in which changes of tone play an essential part (rigidity, tremor, Parkinson's disease).

A unilateral lesion of the substantia nigra is accompanied by similar disorders restricted to the opposite side of the body (unilateral Parkinson's disease).

This coincidence occurs only in two circumstances:

1. In case of lesions of the motor path with severe motor disorders, as occurs in spasmodic hemiplegia or poliomyelitis.
2. In case of grave general condition and rapid development of the disease (cerebral haemorrhage, rapidly developing lethargic encephalitis).

These complex cases being excluded, we observed neither among our material nor in the medical literature, any contradictory case. Thus it is probable that the substantia nigra is one of the mesencephalic regulatory centres of muscle tone. It is not impossible that it may be a sympathetic regulatory centre for tone.

These ideas concern a whole group of clinical phenomena in which tone disorders are a common factor. Paralysis agitans is a specific case in point, in which the relationships between the principal clinical phenomena and the lesions of the substantia nigra are particularly obvious for:

1. In 9 cases of typical paralysis agitans which we examined, degenerative lesions of the substantia nigra seemed absolutely constant and bilateral.

2. In a case of the unilateral form of paralysis agitans, the substantia nigra was affected on the opposite side.

3. In the cases of unilateral, or even monoplegic paralysis agitans published by Blocq and Marinesco, Mendel and Bechet, the substantia nigra showed changes on the opposite side.

4. Finally, we constantly observed lesions of the substantia nigra in diseases such as catatonic paralysis agitans, encephalitis lethargica with catatonia, senile tremor, and diseases with intentional tremor. However, in these various diseases the principal Parkinsonian phenomena of rigidity and tremor are observed in a somewhat isolated fashion. All these findings induce us to conclude that paralysis agitans with its principal symptoms of rigidity and tremor is due to a destructive lesion of the Locus Niger of Soemmering [substantia nigra].

Selected References

Bechet–*Formes cliniques et diagnostic.* Th. de Paris, 1892.
Blocq et Marinesco–Soc. de Biologie, 17 et 25 mai 1893.
Brissaud–*Leçons cliniques sur le mal. nerveuses,* Paris, 1895, leçons 22 et 23.
Hunt–*Atrophic progressive deglobus pallidus* (Brain, vol. XI. part 1, p. 5.).
Ielgersma–*Neue ant. Befunde bei paral. agit. u. Chorea chron.* (Neurol. Zentralblatt 1908).
Lewy–*Zur pathol. Anat. der paral. agitans,* (Neurol. Zentralblatt, 1913, Bd. XXXII, S. 1305).
Mendel–Berliner Klinische Wochenschrift, 1805, no. 29.
Parkinson–*Essay on the Shaking Palsy,* 1817.

Part 4

Chemistry

Levodopa is the generic name for the laevo-optical stereo-isomer of dopa which is the short name for the amino-acid dihydroxy-phenylalanine. L-dopa is the natural form of the main amino acid which is widely distributed in nature both in animals and vegetables.

The first determination of the structure and absolute configuration of levodopa was made by Guggenheim in Basle, Switzerland, in 1913 (Guggenheim M., Z. Physiol. Chem., **88**, *276 1913). He was also the first to undertake a human study for he ingested* 2.5 *g to determine the excretion pattern. A translation of his paper is attached.*

Levodopa can be produced by three main methods: extraction from plant sources, synthesis from vanillin, and from L-tyrosine, but it is these two latter processes that account for the majority of the levodopa in therapeutic use.

In man levodopa is readily and rapidly absorbed following oral administration and peak blood levels are achieved after about two hours. The rate of absorption and blood levels attained depend on several factors including gastric acidity, the rate of gastric emptying and the presence of food.

On the basis of animal experiments it appears that levodopa is widely distributed in the body, particularly in the liver, kidney, gut and skin, with only a small uptake into the brain; and within the brain there is a preferential uptake in the corpus striatum. As judged by cerebro-spinal fluid estimations there is a delay of two to three hours in achieving maximum brain penetration (Pletscher A., Bartholini G., and Tissot R., Brain Research, **4**, *106, 1967).*

The main route of levodopa excretion was originally shown by Guggenheim and is via the urine. Some 80% is recovered in 24 hours, of which over half is in the form of homovanillic acid. The overall metabolism of levodopa is considered in more detail in Part 11.

*Reprinted from M. Guggenheim, Z. Physiol. Chem., **88**, 276, 1913*

DIOXYPHENYLALANINE, A NEW AMINO ACID FROM *VICIA FABA*

M. GUGGENHEIM
HOFFMAN-LA ROCHE, BASLE

As previously pointed out in a collective review[1], adrenaline can be classed as a proteinogenic amine if one takes as its parent substance the hypothetical 3,4-dioxyphenyl-α-methylamino-β-oxypropionic acid. I was therefore greatly interested when, a short while ago,

$$CHOH \cdot CH(NH \cdot CH_3)COOH$$

Torquato Torquati[2] reported that the pods and beans of *Vicia faba* contained a nitrogenous substance which gave a pyrocatechol reaction. The properties of this substance gave reason to suppose that it was closely related to the postulated parent substance of adrenaline.

Largely following the information given by Torquati, I succeeded in obtaining a fairly large quantity of the above substance in crystalline form. A thorough chemical investigation then showed that the isolated nitrogenous pyrocatechol derivative was in all probability 3,4-dioxyphenyl-α-amino propionic acid.

OH

OH

CH$_2$ · CH(NH$_2$) · COOH

This is supported by the elementary analysis, the results of which, while differing slightly from those obtained by Torquati, strongly suggest the formula $C_9H_{11}O_4N$. The presence of two hydroxy groups in the *o*-position can be inferred from the FeCl$_3$ reaction and from the compound's behaviour in respect of heavy-metal salts. Conversion to protocatechuic acid showed that the side chain was in the *p*-position. The optical activity of the compound and the identity of the nitrogen numbers obtained by van Slyke's and Kjeldahl's methods indicate the presence of an amino group. It was also possible to prepare tribenzoyl and tribromide derivatives, the latter crystallizing well.

Dioxyphenylalanine has not previously been found in nature, but the substance has been synthesized by Casimir Funk[3]. The data obtained by the latter author are fairly consistent with our own findings. The melting point of his substance was somewhat lower than that of ours (263–270 °C as opposed to 280 °C), but this is easily explained by the fact that in his case the substance was in the *dl*-form whereas in nature it occurs in the *l*-form. The aim of the present investigations was to adduce final proof of the assumed formula by synthesizing the product, splitting it into its two optically active components and comparing it with the natural substance.

The discovery of a new amino acid is extremely interesting from many points of view. It furnishes proof that amino acids very closely related to our postulated parent substance really do occur in nature. On the other hand, we should always remember that the amino acids so far isolated by no means account for all the possible "building blocks" of amino acids. In fact, some of the biologically most important may yet remain to be discovered. Anyone who has performed acid hydrolysis of a protein will know that it is seldom possible to isolate more than 50–60% of the quantity of amino acids theoretically present. A large part often remains as an indefinable melanin-like residue, still more is lost in other ways as a result of the isolation process. Perhaps this portion contains the very amino acids that are sensitive and unable to withstand the agents used. Dioxyphenylalanine itself, for example, cannot survive the effects of acid hydrolysis. The air and the acid transform it into a black, sparingly soluble pigment.

Dioxyphenylalanine is not fully absorbed in the animal body. In tests on myself and on rabbits I discovered that some of the amino acid is oxidized to protocatechuic acid and some seems to be excreted unchanged.

We still do not know whether this amino acid occurs naturally in the animal body. Nor do we know whether it is used in the synthesis of protein or whether, unlike peptides, it is found only in the free unbound state. These are all questions which must be clarified by further investigation.

At all events, these findings will perhaps encourage a continuing search for new unstable amino acids in the various types of tissue protein. More particularly they will show that we cannot in future afford to ignore the melanin- and resin-like by-products of acid hydrolysis.

Experimental

In principle, the dioxyphenylaminopropionic acid was isolated by Torquati's method (*loc. cit.*). It was based on the insolubility of the substance's lead compound in ammonia solution. 10 kg of *Vicia faba* pods (without the beans) were treated with dilute sulphurous acid and then finely ground in a mincer. This pretreatment with sulphurous acid was designed to prevent the oxidation which would otherwise have occurred very quickly on contact with the iron components of the mincing machine. The ground bean pods were strongly acidified with acetic acid and extracted with about 30 l of water. The cloudy, pale green filtrate was mixed with 2.5 l of 20% lead acetate solution. The abundant precipitate, which settled well, was filtered off and washed. It contained little or no dioxyphenylalanine. The filtrate was made strongly alkaline with ammonia, which yielded an abundant, yellowish-white precipitate. The latter was drawn off and washed several times with water. It was then suspended in about 5 l of water and mixed with hydrogen sulphide. The pale yellow material was separated from the lead sulphide by filtration and concentrated in a current of hydrogen or carbon dioxide at a pressure of about 15 mm. The dioxyphenylalanine separated off as a yellowish-white, crystalline powder. The yield was quite considerable (about 25 g from 10 kg fresh pods). Further, small quantities of the substance were isolated from the mother liquor by renewed precipitation with lead acetate.

For the purposes of purification, the crude amino acid was dissolved in hot water, to which a small quantity of sulphurous acid had been added, and recrystallized in the presence of a little animal charcoal. Depending on the crystallization conditions, the substance finally took the form of well-proportioned, firm prisms or fine needles. Heated in a capillary tube, it decomposed at 280 °C (uncorrected)

Analyses

I 0.1385 g of the substance yielded 0.0679 g H_2O and 0.2745 g CO_2

II 0.1319 g of the substance yielded 0.0661 g H_2O and 0.2612 g CO_2

III 0.115 g of the substance, treated by van Slyke's method at a pressure of 740 mm and a temperature of 24 °C, yielded 14.6 cc N_2

IV 0.2016 g of the substance, treated by Kjeldahl's method, required 10.2 ml O.I N H_2SO_4

Calculated		*Found*			
for $C_9H_{11}O_4N$ (197.12)	I	II	III	IV
C = 54.79%	C = 54.06%	54.01%	—	—
H = 5.62%	H = 5.63%	5.62%	—	—
N = 7.12%	N = —	- -	6.90%	7.09%

For optical determination 1.092 g were dissolved in 10.0450 g normal hydrochloric acid.

$$\frac{20°}{D} \text{ in a 1 dm tube} = -1.40°$$

$$[\alpha]\frac{20°}{D} = -14.28° \ (1 \ 0.2°)$$

The solubility and precipitation reactions of the substance are partly as described by Torquati. It is sparingly soluble in cold water;

one part dissolves in 200 parts of water at 20 °C. In boiling water the solubility is one part in 40. Once dissolved, the substance is slow to separate out on cooling. It is insoluble in alcohol, in all indifferent solvents and in glacial acetic acid.

It dissolves in soda to give a pale yellow colour. This solution gradually turns red-brown on exposure to the air. If prepared under a current of hydrogen, a solution of the substance in caustic alkali is yellow. This turns red on exposure to the air.

The substance dissolves easily in dilute mineral acids to form salts. Evaporation in a desiccator causes the hydrochloric salt to separate out in the form of firm transparent prisms, which disintegrate over concentrated sulphuric acid or calcium chloride.

No picrate could be obtained.

An aqueous solution of this amino acid gives no precipitation with $HgCl_2$. The addition of soda to the mixture, however, yields a brown flocculent precipitate. Neutral lead acetate gives a white flocculent precipitate on the addition of ammonia. Silver nitrate is reduced immediately, without heating. A fairly concentrated solution of iron chloride ($1-5\%$) produces a beautiful and long-lasting emerald-green colour change. A dilute iron chloride solution (0.1%) gives only a transient green colour change; the addition of more iron chloride after this will no longer produce a lasting colour change.

When boiled with copper carbonate the latter passes into solution, liberating CO_2. This solution is bright blue at first but soon becomes darker; evaporation causes oxidation, so no crystallized copper salt can be obtained. Metallic copper powder also dissolves when boiled over a period of time.

Millon's reagent causes an orange-red colour change, diazobenzene sulphonic acid a deep red-brown one. Phosphotungstic acid gives no precipitation; the solution gradually turns red-violet.

When boiled with five times its quantity of saturated alcohol and hydrochloric acid under a current of CO_2, the substance passes into solution. Evaporation in a desiccator gives dioxyphenylalanine hydrochloride in the form of a pink-violet, extremely hygroscopic syrup which is sparingly soluble in ether and easily soluble in alcohol.

Conversion to protocatechuic acid

0.5 g of the substance was added to 5 g of molten caustic alkali.

The latter turned bright yellow and ammonia was vigorously liberated. The mixture was heated until no more gas was given off, taken up in water, acidified and extracted with ether. This left a crystalline residue which, after recrystallization with water, melted at 195 °C.

With iron chloride the substance produced a green colour change, turning to red on the addition of soda.

Tribromodioxyphenylalanine

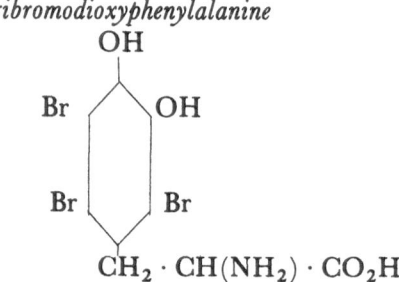

1 g of the substance was placed in a desiccator next to a dish containing bromine in a bell jar. After fairly long exposure to bromine vapour it turned violet, then became white again, and finally deliquesced into a yellowish syrup. This was taken up in sulphurous acid, made weakly alkaline with soda and then acidified with acetic acid. This yielded an abundant quantity of finely interwoven, colourless needles which melted and decomposed at about 200 °C (uncorrected) and contained bromine and nitrogen; these needles were sparingly soluble in cold water and easily soluble in hot. Added to an aqueous solution $FeCl_3$ causes a green colour change which quickly turns to deep blue. After drying at 100 °C, 0.2846 g gave 0.3680 g AgBr in Carius' test.

Calculated for $C_9H_9O_4NBr_3$ (434.0)	Found
Br = 55.27%	Br = 55.30%

Thus, the substance found was evidently a tribromide substitution product.

If iodine is added to an alkaline solution of the amino acid and shaken, a black amorphous pigment which is sparingly soluble in water, immediately separates out.

Tribenzoyldioxyphenylalanine

$$O \cdot OC \cdot C_6H_5$$

$$O \cdot OC \cdot C_6H_5$$

$$CH_2 \cdot CH(NH \cdot CO \cdot C_6H_5) \cdot CO_2H$$

To obtain a benzoyl product of dioxyphenylalanine, the substance was benzoylated in a bicarbonate solution (E. Fischer's method[4]). 1 g of dioxyphenylalanine was suspended in 200 ml of 10% bicarbonate solution and shaken with 6.3 g benzoyl chloride until the smell had dissipated. This gave a voluminous, amorphous, white precipitate, which was dried, dissolved in a little glacial acetic acid and re-precipitated in water. Fine, white needles were obtained whose melting point was in the region of 170 °C. These were sparingly soluble in hot water but easily soluble in glacial acetic acid and alcohol.

0.4250 g, in Kjeldahl's test, required 8.8 ml 0.1 N H_2SO_4.

Calculated for $C_{30}H_{23}O_7N$ (509.17)	Found
N = 2.75%	N = 2.90%

Saponification and a red colour change occur on boiling with an alkali.

Animal experiments

1 g of the substance was administered orally to a rabbit weighing 2200 g. The animal exhibited no unusual symptoms. Its urine was mixed with 20% lead acetate and filtered. The filtrate was made alkaline and the flocculent precipitate was mixed with hydrogen sulphide. An ether-soluble substance was extracted from the concentrated solution and gave a great colour change when mixed with iron chloride. There remained in the aqueous mother liquor an ether-insoluble substance, which also gave a positive pyrocatechol reaction.

Another experiment, in which I myself took $2\frac{1}{2}$ g of the amino acid, yielded similar results. However, in this case I discovered that the substance was not entirely without adverse effects. After about

10 minutes I experienced a feeling of extreme nausea and had to vomit twice. The substance was therefore only partially absorbed.

My urine was tested in the same way as the rabbit's and gave essentially the same results. However, the reaction of iron chloride with urine passed after 5 hours differed from that observed after 2 hours. The 2-hour sample turned green, as was expected, on the addition of iron chloride. The 5-hour urine gradually became darker in neutral and weakly acidic solutions, whereas in ammonia solutions a beautiful blue colour change occurred, this gradually fading to violet.

Like all other known amino acids, dioxyphenylalanine is not very active from the pharmacological point of view. 200 mg administered to a rabbit by intravenous injection caused no significant changes in blood pressure or respiration. Likewise, dioxyphenylalanine has no effect on intact smooth-muscle organs (uterus, intestines).

References

1. Guggenheim, M.: Therap.Monatsch. Vol. 27 (1913): In this paper the hypothetical amino acid was designated as 1,2-dioxyphenyl-4-α-methyl-propionic acid. Here I follow the practice of previous authors in numbering the substituents from the aliphatic side chain.
2. Torquati, Torquato: *On the presence of a nitrogenous substance in the beans of Vicia faba.* Arch. di farmacol, sperim. Vol. 15, pp. 213–23.
   Torquati, Torquato: *On the presence of a nitrogenous substance in the green pods of Vicia faba.* Arch. di farmacol. spermientale, Vol. 15 (1913), pp. 308–12.
3. Funk, Casimir: *Synthesis of d,1–3,4–Dioxyphenylalanine.* Journ. Chem. Soc., London, Vol. 99, pp. 445–57.
4. Fischer, E.: Ber. d. Deutsch. chem. Ges., Vol. 32 (1899), p. 2451.

Part 5

The Recognition of an Action
of Dopamine in the Brain

Although the structure and absolute chemical configuration of levodopa had been determined in 1913 and dopamine, one of its metabolites was known to be widespread thoughout the body, including the brain, it was not until the mid 1950s that the functional significance of dopamine was appreciated. Prior to this it was regarded simply as a precursor of noradrenaline.

Like so much of our recent biochemical and pharmacological knowledge of the central nervous system, the interest in dopamine stemmed from therapeutic and experimental studies on the Rauwolfia alkaloid, reserpine. This substance was found to produce Parkinsonism in man at therapeutic doses and to deplete the tissues of both catecholamines and serotonin.

However, both Blaschko (Blaschko H., Experientia, 13, 9 1957) and Carlsson (Carlsson A., Lindquist M., and Magnusson T., Nature 180, 1200, 1957) suggested in 1957 that the central effects of reserpine might be explained on the basis of dopamine depletion which might have a central role of its own.

The paper by Carlsson and his co-workers has been selected because it compares the effects of both dopa (DL) and 5-hydroxytryptophan in animals pre-treated with reserpine. These amino acid precursors were used because their amine metabolites do not pass the blood-brain barrier. It is interesting to note that the improvement of brain function which was observed with dopa, was potentiated by the simultaneous administration of 5-hydroxytryptophan.

*Reprinted from A. Carlsson, et. al., Nature, **180**, 1200, 1957 by kind permission of the authors and MacMillan Journals Ltd.*

3,4-DIHYDROXYPHENYLALANINE AND 5-HYDROXYTRYPTOPHAN AS RESERPINE ANTAGONISTS

A. CARLSSON, M. LINDQVIST AND T. MAGNUSSON
UNIVERSITY OF LUND

The depletion by reserpine of storage in the body of 5-hydroxy-tryptamine ("serotonin") and of the catechol amines is now well established[1–3]. In reserpinized animals the peripheral part of the adrenergic system does not function owing to lack of the transmitter[2]. This is presumably true also of the central part of the adrenergic system. However, it remains to be proved to what extent the central action of reserpine may be attributed to changes in brain catechol amines and/or 5-hydroxytryptamine.

If lack of amines were responsible for the central action of reserpine, administration of the amines in question should counteract these effects, provided that the amines were capable of entering the brain. However, 5-hydroxytryptamine has been shown not to penetrate the blood-brain barrier readily[4], and this may be true also of the catechol amines. This difficulty may be overcome by administering the amino-acid precursers of the amines. Thus injection of 5-hydroxytryptophan is followed by an increase in the level of 5-hydroxytryptamine in brain as well as central excitation[4]. Preliminary experiments in this laboratory have shown that in this respect 3,4-dihydroxyphenylalanine, which is the precursor of the catechol amines (dopamine, noradrenaline, and adrenaline), behaves similarly.

Experiments were performed on mice (males weighing about 10 gm.), which received an intraperitoneal injection of reserpine (20–40 mgm. per kgm.). After about 16 hr., when the animals were markedly tranquillized and showed complete ptosis of the eyelid, 5-hydroxytryptophan, 3,4-dihydroxyphenylalanine, or a mixture of both amino-acids (in the DL-form throughout) were injected intraperitoneally. In doses up to 1,000 mgm. per kgm. 5-hydroxytryptophan was unable to antagonize the tranquillizing action of reserpine: ptosis persisted. On the other hand, the response to 3,4-dihydroxyphenylalanine was dramatic. Within 15–30 min. after a dose of 500–1,000 mgm. per kgm. the animals resumed almost normal behaviour or even showed signs of overactivity. and ptosis disappeared. The effect did not last much longer than an hour, after which the animals gradually returned to the same condition as before the injection of 3,4-dihydroxyphenylalanine. Although 5-hydroxytryptophan given alone had no effect, a mixture of equal amounts of 5-hydroxytryptophan and 3,4-dihydroxyphenylalanine 250–500 mgm. per kgm.) produced a more complete and longer-lasting counteraction of the reserpine effect than did the same dose of 3,4-dihydroxyphenylalanine alone.

A dramatic effect of 3,4-dihydroxyphenylalanine (200 mgm. per kgm. intravenously) was observed also in rabbits which had received reserpine in a dose of 5 mgm. per kgm. intravenously 4 hr. earlier. Within 10–15 min. after the injection of 3,4-dihydroxyphenylalanine the tranquillization as well as ptosis and meiosis caused by reserpine had disappeared completely. If the animal had received iproniazid (100 mgm. per kgm. intravenously) about 2 hr. before the 3,4-dihydroxyphenylalanine, the dose of the latter required to antagonize the effect of reserpine was markedly reduced. This supports the assumption that the effect of 3,4-dihydroxyphenylalanine was due to an amine formed from it. (The iproniazid, when administered about two hours after the reserpine as in these experiments, did not *per se* counteract the tranquillizing effect of reserpine.) In normal rabbits 3,4-dihydroxyphenylalanine caused central stimulation, which was likewise markedly potentiated by iproniazid pretreatment.

A full account of these experiments will be published elsewhere.

References

1. Shore, P. A. – Pletscher, A. – Tomich, E. G. – Carlsson, A. – Kuntzman, R. – and Brodie, B. B.: *Ann. N.Y. Acad., Sci.,* 66, 609 (1957).
2. Carlsson, A. – Rosengren, E. – Bertler, A. – Nilsson, J.: Internat. Symp. on Psychotropic Drugs, May 9–11, 1957 (in the press).
3. Shore, P. A. – Brodie, B. B.: Internat. Symp. on Psychotropic Drugs, May 9–11, 1057 (in the press).
4. Udenfriend, S. – Weissbach, H. – Bogdanski, D. F.: *Ann. N.Y. Acad. Sci.,* 66, 602 (1957).

Part 6

Pathophysiological Findings in Parkinsonism

The suggestion that the midbrain area and specifically the substantia nigra were abnormal in Parkinsonism was first made in 1893 and confirmed in the early part of this century (see Section 3). This was followed by the observation that in animals dopa reverses the effects of reserpine.

*In 1960 Ehringer and Hornykiewicz (Klin. Wschr **38**, 1236, 1960) studied the dopamine and noradrenaline levels of various brain areas of seventeen adult subjects, two foetuses and one child. They then compared the results with those obtained in fourteen patients who had exhibited extra-pyramidal symptoms, including four with postencephalitic Parkinsonism, two with idiopathic Parkinsonism, two with Huntington's chorea, plus one case of infantile cerebral damage and five cases with symptoms of unknown cause. The miscellaneous cases showed levels which did not deviate from normal, but in the idiopathic and postencephalitic Parkinsonian patients there was a marked reduction in the normally high levels of dopamine in the corpus striatum but no significant changes in other areas and no consistent changes in adrenaline in any region.*

It was considered that the reduction of the dopamine levels in the corpus striatum could be causative in the genesis of the Parkinsonian syndrome. This hypothesis had exciting therapeutic implications.

*This work has since been extended. Thus, for example, Hornykiewicz (Hornykiewicz O., Pharmac. Rev., **18**, 925, 1966) has reviewed the whole subject up to 1965. More recently the subject has been reviewed again by Moore (Moore R. Y., in l-Dopa and Parkinsonism, Ed. Barbeau A., McDowell F. H., F. A. Davis Co., 1970, p. 143) who has also demonstrated* *directly the presence of a nigro-striatal pathway by the technique of anterograde degeneration.*

The current pathophysiological situation pertaining to Parkinson's disease may be summarised as :

(a) Degeneration of melanin-containing nerve cells of the pars compacta of the substantia nigra.

(b) Depleted dopamine levels in the striatal region of Parkinsonism patients with low urinary dopamine excretion, but normal homovanillic acid excretion in the urine. The striatal dopamine deficiency is well correlated with the extent of the cell loss of the pars compacta of the substantia nigra and in hemi-Parkinsonism the dopamine depletion is more pronounced on the contralateral side to the symptoms.

(c) In animals, substantia nigral ablation depletes striatal dopamine. Stimulation of the substantia nigra leads to an increase of dopamine collected from a cannula inserted in the putamen.

(d) Inhibition of caudate neurons has followed stimulation of the substantia nigra and the application of dopamine to neurons in the caudate nucleus has shown inhibition in the majority of cells.

Translated from H. Ehringer and O. Hornykiewicz, Wien. Klin. Wschr., **38**, 1236, *1960, by kind permission of the authors and Springer-Verlag*

DISTRIBUTION OF NORADRENALINE AND DOPAMINE (3-HYDROXYTYRAMINE) IN THE HUMAN BRAIN AND THEIR BEHAVIOUR IN THE PRESENCE OF DISEASE AFFECTING THE EXTRA-PYRAMIDAL SYSTEM

H. EHRINGER AND O. HORNYKIEWICZ
UNIVERSITY OF VIENNA

It is known that catecholamines are present in the brain of mammals (v. Euler; Holtz (1950). In a fundamental study of localisation of sympathin, which is a mixture of noradrenaline and adrenaline, Vogt (1951) was able to demonstrate that in the brain of dogs the concentration in the various parts of the brain does not coincide with the vascular supply, i.e. the amount of sympathetic vascular nerves. The greatest quantity of sympathin is found in certain function centres, especially in the areas of the central representation of the sympathetic nervous system, viz.: in the hypothalamus, in the stratum griseum centrale and in the sympathetic centres of the medulla oblongata. However, the physiological significance of sympathin in these structures is not yet completely clear, especially because 5-hydroxytryptamine is abundantly present there as well. Recently, a third catecholamine, 3,4-dihydroxyphenylethylamine (3-hydroxytyramine = dopamine) has assumed importance, which had already for a long time been considered as the precursor of noradrenaline (Demis, Blaschko and Welch 1955; Hagen and Welch, 1955; Hagen 1956). Dopamine also was soon demonstrated in the human brain and in the brain of various mammals (Montagu 1957; Carlsson, Lindquist, Magnusson, Waldeck 1958).

It is extremely interesting that Bertler and Rosengren (1959) observed the highest dopamine content in the corpus striatum. However, here there is only little noradrenaline and 5-HT. This striking distribution suggests that dopamine in addition to its significance as precursor of noradrenaline, also plays an inherent physiological part in the function of these nuclei. If in fact noradrenaline and dopamine play a specific part in brain function, then a change of concentration of these substances would cause a change of function in the affected areas. As far as we know, no changes of the catecholamine content in the presence of disease affecting the human brain, especially the extrapyramidal system, have ever been described. Birkmayer advised us to carry out post mortem studies of the 5-HT content of the hypothalamus of patients with Parkinson's disease. In this disease there are functional disorders in the ganglia of the extrapyramidal system, where Bartler and Rosengren had found particularly high concentrations of dopamine. As in a small piece of tissue we were unable to estimate at the same time shall amounts of 5-HT, dopamine and noradrenaline, we could only study dopamine and noradrenaline in certain cerebral regions.

The purpose of this investigation was:

1. To estimate in the normal human brain the dopamine and noradrenaline content of the various regions. For this purpose, we studied post mortem the brains of neurologically normal patients.

2. Determination of the catecholamine in the developing human brain; for this we studied the brains of two foetuses.

3. Study of the brains of patients with extrapyramidal manifestations. Among these there were 4 cases of postencephalitic Parkinsonism, 2 cases of Parkinson's disease (paralysis agitans), 2 cases of Huntington's chorea and various other illnesses that were accompanied by extrapyramidal symptoms.

Method and material

These investigations have been carried out in human brains, which we obtained by courtesy of the Institute of Patho-anatomy of the University of Vienna and from the hospital of the City of Vienna-Lainz.

The brains were dissected 3–20 h after death, in the following way: several frontal cuts were made through the brain, so that the brain slices obtained provided good orientation which permitted easy preparation of the various regions and nuclei. During the delimitation of the nuclei, care was taken to exclude any white substance. This material which was not fixed was immediately placed into hermetically sealed test tubes and cooled to $-20°$C, the material being thawed out again just before the examination. The extraction of noradrenaline and dopamine was carried out according to the method of Beetler, Carlsson and Rosengren (1958), by means of perchloric acid and by using an ion exchanger Dowex 50×8 (200–400 mesh) with the modifications described by Holzer and Hornykiewicz (1959). The elution of noradrenaline was carried out with 6 ml 1 N HCl; the elution of dopamine was carried out with 6 ml 2 N HCl. The quantitative estimation of noradrenaline was carried out by a modification described by Sharpdryer (1958) of the fluorimetric method of v. Euler and Floding (1956). The noradrenalineinates were brought with $NaHCO_3$ (substance) a pH of 3–4 and the oxidation was carried out with an acetate buffer at pH 6. With this pH the sum of adrenaline and noradrenaline are demonstrated. As with this method by oxidation at pH 3.5 we were never able to demonstrate adrenaline in the human brain, we subsequently defined as "noradrenaline" the figures obtained at pH 6. The measurements were carried out in a Beckman photofluorimeter by using a quinine standard (0.25μg/ml in 0.1 N H_2SO_4) and Schott GB 12 filter as entrance filter and Schott OG 4 as exit filter. The dopamine fraction (2 N HCl) was dried *in vacuo* at 55–60 °C, the residue was absorbed in 1 ml distilled water and estimated quantitatively by the colorimetric method of v. Euler and Hamberg (1949) at 529μm. The sensitivity of this method of about 2μg is limited, when as blank figure the non-oxidised extract is considered. The relatively low sensitivity of this method compelled us, in the case of areas of small weight and presumably low dopamine content, to collect the material from several brains to carry out the test. This procedure permitted us to determine also relatively low figures per gramme tissue. In some areas the mean figures were estimated only in this way.

Results

1. *Distribution of noradrenaline and dopamine in the brain of adult human beings*
The results obtained in 17 adult brains are shown in Table 1.

Table 1. — Levels of noradrenaline and dopamine in brain nuclei of "normals"

Brain area	Noradrenaline (μg/g wt.)			Dopamine (μg/g wt.)		
	Number of brains examined*	Range	Mean	Number of brains examined*	Range	Mean
Telencephalon						
Nucl. caudatus	6	0.06–0.14	0.09	10	2.7–5.5	3.5
Putamen	7	0.08–0.14	0.12	12	2.1–5.3	3.7
Globus pallidus	7 (4)	0.05–0.30	0.15	13 (6)	0.8–1.8	0.5
Nucl. amygdala	7 (3)	0.08–0.24	0.21	5 (2)	0.5–1.0	0.6
Septum region	4 (1)	—	0.31	4 (1)	—	0.3
Substantia alba	1	—	0.01	1	—	0.0
Diencephalon						
Thalamus	5 (3)	0.09–0.14	0.13	8 (4)	0.2–0.4	0.3
Thalamus (medial)	3 (1)	—	0.22	3 (1)	—	0.4
Hypothalamus	11 (5)	0.80–1.67	1.25	11 (5)	0.5–1.7	0.8
Mesencephalon						
Nucl. ruber	7 (2)	0.29–0.40	0.30	9 (2)	0.5–1.1	0.7
Stratum griseum cent.	6 (1)	—	0.46	6 (1)	—	0.5
Pretectal region	5 (1)	—	0.12	5 (1)	—	0.4
Substantia nigra	8 (2)	0.20–0.28	0.21	7 (1)	—	0.9
Rhombencephalon						
Formatio reticularis	8 (3)	0.23–0.34	0.28	5 (2)	0.3–0.6	0.6
Ventricular	7 (2)	0.29–0.39	0.35	12 (3)	0.2–1.0	0.6
Nucl. olivarum	4 (1)	—	0.11	7 (2)	0.4–0.8	0.6
Pons	2 (1)	—	0.13	2 (1)	—	0.2
Area postrema	3 (1)	—	2.00	3 (1)	—	1.3
Cerebellum						
Nucl. dentatus	4 (1)	—	0.06	4 (1)	—	<0.5

*The number of brains examined individually is shown in brackets. The others were pooled and average values taken.

The distribution of noradrenaline in our material is largely similar to the figures reported by Vogt (1951) for sympathin in the brain of dogs. Sano, Gamo, Kakimoto, Taniguchi, Takesada and Nishinuma (1959) obtained similar results for noradrenaline in three human brains (poisoning, strangulation, cerebral embolism) and for dopamine (see also Bertler and Rosenberg 1959a). The consistency of our results is remarkable: there was but little difference in the amine concentration, independently of whether the brains were dissected and frozen three or 20 hours after death. This made it possible to compare these figures with those of other brains, which had been studied under the same conditions.

2. *Distribution of noradrenaline and dopamine in the various areas of the brain of human foetuses.*

The brain of a 48 cm long and that of a 40 cm long human foetus was studied. We extracted only the areas that could definitely be differentiated. The results are summarised in Table 2.

It is noteworthy that in all the areas studied, and particularly in the hypothalamus, the noradrenaline content was already in the range of normal, whereas the dopamine content of the corpus striatum was definitely lower than in normal adults. In contrast, both the figures for dopamine and noradrenaline in the brain of a child aged four months correspond to the comparative figures in Table 2.

Table 2.—Noradrenaline and dopamine in selected brain areas of foetuses

Brain area	Noradrenaline (μg/g wt.)		Dopamine (μg/g wt.)	
	Foetus 48 cm long	Foetus 40 cm long	Foetus 48 cm long	Foetus 40 cm long
Nucl. caudatus	0.14	not studied	0.3	not studied
Putamen	0.15	0.12	1.0	1.1
Globus pallidus	0.32	0.35	—	not studied
Hypothalamus	1.16	0.92	—	not studied

3. *Dopamine and noradrenaline in the brains of patients suffering from extrapyramidal disorders.*

In order to obtain possible indications as to the physiological function of dopamine and noradrenaline in the central nervous system, we carried out a post-mortem study of the brains of 14 patients who had shown extrapyramidal symptoms. Some of these patients also showed autonomic symptoms.

(a) *Postencephalitic Parkinsonism*

For the diagnosis of this syndrome, there was encephalitis in the past history, oculogyric crisis, extrapyramidal and autonomic manifestations as well as decolouration of the substantia nigra, as valid criteria. The noradrenaline and dopamine concentration in the important brain areas of four such cases are shown in Table 3. The

51

Table 3.—Noradrenaline and dopamine in postencephalitic Parkinsonism

Brain area	Noradrenaline (µg/g wt.)		Dopamine (µg/g wt.)	
	Individual results	Mean	Individual results	Mean
Nucl. caudatus	0.00–0.02–0.04–0.00	0.02	0.1–0.3–0.0–0.5	0.2
Putamen	0.01–0.02–0.05–0.04	0.03	0.3–0.5–0.2–0.1	0.3
Globus pallidus	0.46–0.13–0.20–0.14	0.23	0.1–0.2–0.0 —	0.1
Hypothalamus	— 0.27–1.99–0.68	0.98	not studied	

other areas which we studied, showed no notable changes in comparison with normal, and they are not considered in the table.

In this disease, the markedly low dopamine levels are particularly noteworthy in the nucleus caudatus and in the putamen. In two of these cases, also the noradrenaline content of the hypothalamus was reduced. We again should like to emphasise that the brains were examined under identical conditions as those comparative brains in Table 1.

(b) *Parkinson's disease*
The determining criteria for the diagnosis were the clinical aspect, i.e. the absence of oculogyric episodes, no encephalitis in the past history, as well as late onset of the disease. We were able to study two such cases. The findings are shown in Table 4.

Table 4.—Noradrenaline and dopamine in Parkinson's disease

Brain area	Noradrenaline (µg/g wt.)		Dopamine (µg/g wt.)	
	Individual results	Mean	Individual results	Mean
Nucl. caudatus	0.06–0.10	0.03	1.9–0.3	1.1
Putamen	0.08–0.06	0.07	1.2–0.3	0.8
Globus pallidus	0.06	not studied	0.3	not studied
Hypothalamus	0.53	not studied	not studied	not studied

The important point is that the dopamine level was also obviously reduced in the corpus striatum, but not as much as in the brains of postencephalitic Parkinsonism. In one case, the noradrenaline level was also clearly reduced.

(c) *Other extrapyramidal syndromes*
We also studied two cases of Hungtington's chorea, one case of

infantile cerebral damage and five patients who had shown extra-pyramidal symptoms (tremor, rigidity and hyperkinesia) of unknown origin, as to the catecholamine content of the brains. In none of these cases were we able to determine levels deviating from normal.

Discussion

The findings in this investigation can be classified in three groups: topography of dopamine and noradrenaline in the human brain, behaviour of these two catecholamines during the development of the brain and behaviour of dopamine and noradrenaline in diseases affecting the extrapyramidal system.

Regarding the topography of dopamine in the human brain, we should like to add the following to what we have already stated: as higher concentrations of dopamine are found only in the neostriatum, it is very likely that it exerts a special function in these ganglia. The high dopamine content of the nucleus caudatus and putamen is surprising, when one considers that Undenfriend and Creveling (1959) were able to demonstrate an equally great dopamine-β-oxidase activity here as in the hypothalamus; this enzyme is responsible for the hydroxylation of dopamine into noradrenaline. However, as the neostriatum is very poor in noradrenaline one must assume that in the neostriatum, dopamine and the hydroxylating enzyme are contained in different cell elements, so that dopamine is protected against the action of the enzyme.

The opposite behaviour of dopamine and of noradrenaline during the embryonic development of the brain is very interesting. Whereas the dopamine content of the neostriatum was obviously lower in the foetuses which we studied, than in adults, in these cases the noradrenaline content of the hypothalamus was already almost completely normal. These findings may perhaps be explained by what is known about the embryonic development of the brain. According to Spatz (1925), the diencephalon attains a fairly high degree of maturity already at the end of the third month, whereas the neostriatum becomes differentiated much later. Thus it is possible that in the less differentiated cells and tissues also the activity of the necessary enzymes for the synthesis and breakdown of the catecholamines is correspondingly lower than in structures, the maturity of which is already more advanced. Shimizu and

Morikawa (1969) demonstrated such differences in the activity of monoamine oxidase in the developing brain of rats. We have no knowledge of similar investigations regarding the enzymes that play an important part in the catecholamine metabolism.

The cases of Parkinson's disease and postencephalitic Parkinsonism which we studied indicated a dopamine content reduced to about one-tenth in the neostriatum. All these cases presented an akinetic hypertonic syndrome: akinesia accompanied by rigidity and slight resting tremor. In contrast, in extrapyramidal syndromes of the hyperkinetic type such as Hungtington's chorea, the investigations showed a normal dopamine content. It seems logical to relate the akinetic hypertonic symptoms to the deficiency of dopamine in the neostriatum. However, whether these can be attributed to the low dopamine content, could not be demonstrated in our investigations.

To try to obtain confirmation of this by means of animal experiments is very difficult, because the experimentally-induced reduction of dopamine is always accompanied by a reduction also of the noradrenaline and 5-HT level. In this respect, perhaps the development of Parkinson-like manifestations after prolonged treatment with reserpine indicate to a certain extent an analogy to our findings; among other things reserpine reduces the dopamine level in the brain (Carlsson, Lindquist, Magnusson and Waldeck, 1958). In effect, according to Carlsson, Lindquist and Magnusson (1957), certain effects of reserpine (namely sedation) can be neutralised in animals by Dopa, which is a precursor of noradrenaline and dopamine. There could be a similar explanation for the long-known effect that using harmaline alkaloids (which also raise the dopamine content in the brain (Holzer and Hornykiewicz 1959) good results have also been obtained in Parkinson's disease (Gunn 1935). However, it is certain that regarding dopamine, we could not find any fundamental difference between postencephalitic Parkinsonism and Parkinson's disease; the biochemical changes, however, were more marked in postencephalitic Parkinsonism. This is in agreement with the concept of Klaub (1940) regarding the pathogenesis of these two syndromes.

On the basis of our findings, we should like briefly to discuss the question of the localisation of the brain dopamine. Whereas dopamine in the periphery is partly localised in defined chromaffin cells (Bertler, Falk, Hillarp, Rosengren and Torp 1959; Eade 1958), nothing is known of its localisation in the cells of the neostriatum. In principle, three types of cells may be considered; small ganglionic cells which are much more numerous; great multipolar (polygonal) ganglionic cells of which there are fewer and finally, glia cells. Regarding this question, based on our investigations we should like to conjecture as follows: according to data in the literature (Haller-Vorden 1957), in Huntington's chorea there is a deficiency of up to 90% of small cells in the neostriatum and a moderate glia proliferation; in spite of this, and in accordance with our findings, the dopamine content of these nuclei is practically normal. Thus, the ganglia cells are probably not the site of dopamine and there remain the large ganglionic cells and the glia. Of these two types of cells, we are inclined to give preference to the multipolar cells. However, in order to obtain evidence of this, one would have to study diseases in which this type of cell is selectively affected. However, according to experience, in Parkinson's disease and postencephalitic Parkinsonism, only insignificant histological changes can be demonstrated in the neostriatum and from these one hardly can draw any definite conclusions. Thus it appears that in these two diseases, it is mainly a question of functional changes of the cells in the neostriatum, related perhaps to the dopamine metabolism.

The great reduction of dopamine in the neostriatum of subjects with Parkinson's disease and postencephalitic Parkinsonism, is apart from the findings of Bertler and Rosenberg (1950), nevertheless a new indication of the physiological importance of dopamine in these nuclei. Unfortunately, we were able to study only six such cases. Should this finding be confirmed in further cases, one could consider it as important as the changes in the substantia nigra. In this case, dopamine would play a particularly significant part in the symptomatology of Parkinson's disease and postencephalitic Parkinsonism. In addition, this would represent for the first time a direct indication to the physiolocal part played by the cerebral dopamine.

The reduction of noradrenaline in the hypothalamus of three cases could very likely be due to the cell deficiency observed in this area.

References

Bertler, A. – Carlsson, A. – Rosengren, E.: Fysiogr. Sällsk. Handl. *28*, 121, 1958.
Bertler, A. – Falk, B. – Hillarp, A. – Rosengren, E. – Torp, A.: Acta physiol. Scand., *47*, 251, 1959.
Bertler, A. – Rosengren, E., Experientia (Basel), *15*, 10, 1959.
Bertler, A. – Rosengren, E., Experientia, *15*, 382, 1959a.

Carlsson, A. – Lindquist, M. – Magnusson, T.: Nature (Lund), *180*, 1200, 1957.
Carlsson, A. – Lindquist, M. – Magnusson, T. – Waldeck, B.: Science, *127*, 471, 1958.
Demis, D. J. – Blaschko, H. – Welch, A. D.: J. Pharmacol, *117*, 208, 1955.
Eade, N. R.: J. Physiol. (Lond.), *141*, 183, 1958.
Euler, U. S. v.: Acta physiol. Scand., *12*, 73, 1946.
Euler, U. S. v., u. – Floding, I.: Acta physiol. Scand., *33*, Suppl., 118, 57, 1955.
Euler, U. S. v. – Hamberg, U.: Acta physiol. Scand., *19*, 74, 1949.
Gunn, J. A.: Arch. int. Pharmacodyn., *50*, 379, 1935.
Hagen, P.: J. Pharmacol, *116*, 26, 1956.
Hagen, P. – Welch, A.: Recent. Progr. Hormone Res., *12*, 27, 1955.
Hallervorden, J.: Handbuch der speziellen pathologischen Anatomie und Pathologie, Bd. XIII/I/A, S. 798, 1957.
Holtz, P.: Acta physiol. Scand., *20*, 354, 1950.
Holzer, G. – Hornykiewicz, O.: Naunyn-Schmiedeberg's Arch. exp. Path. Pharmak.,w*37*, 27, 1959.
Montagu, K. A.: Nature (Lond.), *180*, 244, 1957.
Sano, I. – Gamo, T. – Kakimoto, Y. – Taniguchi, K. – Takesada, M. – Nishinuma, K.: Biochem. biophys., Acta, *32*, 586, 1959.
Schaepdryver, A. F. de: Arch. int. Pharmacodyn., *115*, 233, 1958.
Shimizu, N. – Morikawa, N.: Nature (Lond.), *184*, 650, 1959.
Spatz, H.: Anat. Anz., Erg.-Bd., *60*, 54, 1925.
Klauee, R.: Arch. Psychiat. Nervenkr., *111*, 251, 1940.
Udenfriend, S. – Creveling, C. R.: J. Neurochem., *4*, 350, 1959.
Vogt, Marthe: J. Physioll (Lond.), *123*, 451, 1954.
Weil-Malherbe, H. – Bone, A. D.: Nature *180*, 1050, 1957.

Part 7

The Initial Clinical Trials

Hornykiewicz followed up his study of the dopamine content of the brain in Parkinsonism with a collaborative study with Birkmayer of the Neurological Clinic, Vienna, on the therapeutic effects of levodopa. (Birkmayer W., and Hornykiewicz O., Wien. Klin. Wschr. **73**, *787, 1961). They administered single intravenous doses of 50 to 150 mg in saline and showed that it reduced or completely suppressed the akinesia for periods from three to twenty four hours but showed no noticeable effect on the rigidity and tremor. They furthermore noted that intravenous injection of 5-hydroxytryptophan also appeared to have a beneficial effect.*

Quite independently in Montreal, Barbeau and co-workers (Barbeau A., Murphy G. F., and Sourkes T. L., in the Bel-Air Symposium of Monoamines and the Central Nervous System, Georg et Cie, Geneva 1961, p. 247 also demonstrated the value of dopa but used the levo form by the oral route. The dose used, i.e. 100 to 200 mg in acute experiments, was significantly above the quantity of levodopa administered by Birkmayer and Hornykiewicz. They found about 50% reduction in rigidity beginning about thirty minutes after ingestion of the levodopa and persisting for about two hours, but with little effect on tremor. The D-form on the other hand showed no significant effect.

Translations of both these papers are appended.

Translated from W. Birkmayer and O. Hornykiewicz, Wien. Klin. Wschr., **73**, 787, *1961, by kind permission of the authors and Springer-Verlag.*

THE EFFECT OF L-3,4-DIOXYPHENYLALANINE (=DOPA) IN PARKINSONIAN AKINESIA

W. BIRKMAYER AND O. HORNYKIEWICZ
VIENNA-LAINZ CITY HOSPITAL AND UNIVERSITY OF VIENNA

Rigidity, tremor and akinesia are the cardinal symptoms of the Parkinsonian syndrome. Whereas rigidity can be favourably influenced by many drugs, and the tremor can to a certain extent be allayed by compounds with atropine-like action, akinesia has represented so far a therapeutic problem without solution. When six years ago we adopted M. Bleuler's reserpine therapy for chorea, we observed that overdosage led to the development of the Parkinsonian syndrome. As, among other actions, reserpine also releases serotonin (=5-hydroxytryptamine), we subsequently tried to obtain basic information regarding the serotonin metabolism in this disease by estimating the 5-hydroxyindolacetic acid in the urine and CSF of patients suffering from Parkinsonism. This investigation gave a negative result but nevertheless a clinical trial supported our concept that in Parkinsonism there could exist a disorder of serotonin metabolism. We injected a Parkinsonian patient during the oculogyric crisis with 25 mg "Marsilid" (=Iproniazid), a MAO inhibitor, intravenously. Whereas the oculogyric crisis in this patient usually lasted only a few hours, after the injection of "Marsilid" it became dangerously more marked and lasted three days. As both reserpine and "Marsilid" (which affect the metabolism of serotonin and other amines) exerted an obvious influence on the Parkinsonian syndrome, we were convinced of the important part played by these amines in this disease. Already at that time (1958) a study of the behaviour of serotonin in the brain of patients with Parkinsonism had been proposed by one of us (W.B.), but for technical reasons this could not be carried out at that time.

When in 1959 Bertler and Rosengren were able to demonstrate that dopamine (3-hydroxytyramine), which had already been known for some time, was the immediate precursor of noradrenaline and that in the brain of animals it has a very specific distribution, being confined almost exclusively on the nuclei of the neostriatum, one of us (O.H.) proposed the study of the distribution of this amine in the brain of normal subjects and in subjects suffering from Parkinsonism. This proposal was based on the concept that the specific distribution of the dopamine in the centres of the extrapyramidal-motor system could possibly be the expression of a specific function of dopamine in these centres. The Parkinson syndrome with its known disorders of the extrapyramidal system seemed thus especially suited for studying the significance of brain dopamine. In addition to the behaviour of the dopamine, the distribution of noradrenaline and finally also that of serotonin was investigated. These investigations (Ehringer and Hornykiewicz, 1960; Bernheimer, Birkmayer and Hornykeiwicz, 1961) showed that in Parkinsonism (Parkinson's disease, postencephalitic Parkinsonism), the concentration of dopamine, noradrenaline, and serotonin is greatly reduced; especially marked is the reduction of dopamine in the caudate nucleus and in the putamen. In Parkinsonian patients there is also a reduction of dopamine in the urine when compared with control subjects (Barbeau, Murphy and Sourkes 1961).

Based on these results, one of us (O.H.) proposed in a series of trials in Parkinson patients the administration of L-3,4-dioxyphenylalanine (=Dopa) which is the immediate precursor of dopamine. Because it will not pass the blood-brain barrier, dopamine itself hardly penetrates into the brain. However L-Dopa, which easily penetrates the blood-brain barrier, is then readily decarboxylated into dopamine in the brain; in this way we tried to increase the previously reduced dopamine concentration in Parkinson patients. In 1960, Degkwitz, Frowein, Kulenkampff and Hohs administered L-Dopa intravenously to insane and normal subjects and, as was known from animal experiments (Carlsson, Lindquist and Magnusson, 1957), they were able to demonstrate among other things that the sedative effect of reserpine was effectively neutralized by L-Dopa. The authors administered 50 to 350 mg intravenously and the side effects consisted mostly of nausea, tachycardia, sweating, anxiety and vomiting.

Like Degkwitz *et al.*, we diluted L-Dopa in boiling hot saline solution and we injected 50, 100 and 150 mg slowly intravenously. There were both patients with moderately severe and severe post-encephalitic Parkinsonism and Parkinson's disease. In cases of Parkinson's syndrome, the effect of a single intravenous L-Dopa injection consisted mainly of a complete or significant reduction of the akinesia. Patients who previously could not change from a prone position to a sitting position; could not stand up from a sitting position or from a standing position could not start walking, were able to perform all this easily after administration of L-Dopa. Their movements were normal and they were even able to run or jump. The previously aphonic speech with the unclear articulation due to palilalia became, as in normal subjects, strong and clear. For a short time the patients were able to achieve motor performances which previously could not be approached by the use of any other drug. This Dopa effect reached its peak within two to three hours and then persisted in a lesser degree for 24 hours. In some patients, especially in those milder cases, a more fluid spontaneous mobility lasted even longer. So far we have observed this effect in all Parkinson patients whom we have studied (20 cases), but in varying degrees; the effect was slightest in arteriosclerotic Parkinsonism. The Dopa effect depended on the dose; 50 mg produced the slightest and 150 mg the most marked anti-akinetic effect. As side effects of too rapid injection or higher doses, (150 mg) sweating and vomiting occurred.

The blood pressure rose on an average 10 to 20 mm Hg, the heart rate by about 10 beats per minute. An additional injection of 300 mg vitamin B_6 or 1000 mg vitamin C produced no increase of the effect. Pretreatment of the patient with a MAO inhibitor ("Marplan") very obviously increased and prolonged the anti-akinetic effect of L-Dopa. Barbeau and Sourkes (1961) and Barbeau (1961) have found that the Parkinsonian rigidity can be favourably influenced with long-term oral administration of L-Dopa. With our method of a single intravenous dose of L-Dopa we could not observe a significant influence of L-Dopa on the rigidity.

Summary

As a result of investigations carried out by Hornykiewicz *et al.*, who observed an especially marked deficiency of dopamine in the caudate

nucleus and putamen of Parkinson patients, such patients were given
L-Dopa which easily penetrated the blood-brain barrier and which
is the immediate precursor of dopamine. Doses of 50 to 150 mg
were given by intravenous injection. The result consisted of a complete suppression or of reduction of the akinesia. This Dopa effect
lasted for about three hours undiminished, after which it gradually
disappeared, usually over 24 hours. This effect could always be
reproduced with the same dose and degree of effect. According to
our experience up to now, the rigidity and tremor were not notably
influenced by a single dose. The transient suppression of the akinesia
due to the effect of Dopa is undoubtedly the starting point for
rational therapy of this syndrome, if it happens that this effect could
be made to last longer. In this respect, a combination with MAO
inhibitors seems encouraging.

Observations after proof-reading; trials with 5-hydroxytryptophan, the
precursor of serotonin, indicate that in the Parkinson syndrome the
brain serotonin also plays a part that still needs further clarification.
According to our preliminary findings, intravenous injection of
5-hydroxytryptophan also seems to lead to improvement in Parkinsonism.

References

Barbeau, A.: VIIIth International Congress of Neurology, Rome, Sept., 1961.
Barbeau, A. – Murphy, G. F. – Sourkes, T. L.: Science, *133*, (1961), 1706.
Barbeau, A. – Sourkes, T. L.: *Personal communication.*
Bernheimer, H. – Birkmayer, W. – Hornykiewicz, O.: Klin. Wschr., *39*, (1961), 1056.
Bertler, A. – Rosengren, E.: Experientia, *15*, (1959), 10.
Carlsson, A. – Lindquist, M. – Magnusson, T.: Nature, *180*, (1957), 1200.
Degkwitz, R. – Frowein, R. – Kulenkampff, C. – Mohs, U.: Klin. Wschr., *33*, (1969), 120.
Ehringer, H. – Hornykiewicz, O.: Klin. Wschr., *38*, (1960), 1236.

Translated from A. Barbeau, et al., Bel-Air Symposium on Monoamines and the Central Nervous System Geneva 1961, by kind permission of the authors and George et Cie S.A.

CATECHOLAMINES IN PARKINSONISM

A. BARBEAU, T. L. SOURKES AND G. F. MURPHY
UNIVERSITY OF MONTREAL AND THE ALLAN
MEMORIAL INSTITUTE, MONTREAL

The results of several investigations performed in recent years would appear to suggest that abnormal catecholamine (particularly dopamine) metabolism features in certain diseases of the basal ganglia. These investigations were prompted, inter alia, by the observations of Montague[1], who identified dopamine and dopa (3,4-dihydroxyphenylalanine) in the brain, and by the findings of Carlsson, Sano, and Goldstein et al.,[2,3,4,5,6] who demonstrated the special distribution of dopamine in these structures. Using as our basis the analogy of the pharmacological action of reserpine and the induction by this drug of Parkinsonian syndromes, we studied the urinary excretion of catecholamines in certain diseases of the basal ganglia[7,8]. Our results showed that the daily urinary excretion of dopamine was selectively reduced in Parkinson's disease, particularly in the postencephalitic and arteriosclerotic forms[9]. Two other investigations have now confirmed our results. Williams et al.[10] have shown that the excretion of homovanillic acid is reduced in Parkinson's disease, and Ehringer and Hornykiewicz[11] have found considerable reductions in the dopamine and norepinephrine contents of the brains of six patients with Parkinson's disease. These reductions were also more marked in subjects with the postencephalitic form of the disease.

The aim of the present investigations is to extend these observations and to study, in clinical tests, the effect of modifying the dopamine level. We hope that in this way we shall be able to demonstrate

63

the relationship between catecholamines and the symptoms of Parkinson's disease.

Material and Methods

1. Estimations

The estimation of adrenaline and noradrenaline was carried out by the method of trihydroxy indole[12], that of dopamine by a modification of the procedure of Carlsson and Waldeck[12] and that of dopac (dihydroxyphenylacetic acid), after purification on aluminium oxide column, by paper chromatography and fluorescence with ethylene diamine. All these estimations were carried out in 24-hour urines kept in cold storage in the presence of 10 cc of 18% hydrochloric acid.

2. Biochemical and clinical studies

These studies were carried out in 69 patients who were suffering from Parkinson's disease in different stages. Furthermore, 31 individuals of our laboratory staff and 20 schizophrenics at the mental hospital Saint-Jean-de-Dieu served as controls at different stages of the investigation. The following criteria were adopted for classification of the Parkinson cases:

(1) Postencephalitic: history of an episode suggesting encephalitis and the presence of typical oculogyric crises.
(2) Arteriosclerotic: onset of symptoms after 65 years, evidence of generalised arteriosclerosis (typical arterial tension) and predominance of rigidity over the other symptoms.
(3) Idiopathic: the other cases.

We are aware of the fact that these criteria are severe and tend to increase the "idiopathic" group as opposed to the others, but it permits us to compare our cases with those of other authors.

3. Evaluation of the rigidity and tremor

In all patients this was done in two ways. Usually four examiners (and always at least two) made a clinical evaluation of these two symptoms at the level of the head, chin, tongue and each limb. A scale of from + to + + + was used for each part of the body studied. The total of points constituted the clinical score of rigidity or tremor of the patient. This evaluation was carried out every day or on the occasion of each test and change of medication.

In addition, each patient was subjected to a series of physical tests already described previously[13], which are a modification of those already reported by Burns and De Jong[14]. This series of tests consists of fourteen tests for studying the rigidity and three for studying the tremor. Thus, it is possible to obtain a score of performance and a score of tremor.

Results

For the sake of greater clarity, the results will be divided into two parts: biochemical studies and clinical studies.

(a) *Biochemical studies*

1. *Urinary estimation of catecholamines in Parkinson's disease*
The three catecholamines adrenaline, noradrenaline and dopamine were studied in the 24-hour urines of 31 normal subjects and 30 patients suffering from Parkinson's disease. This study includes 2 series of patients. The first 15 cases* has already been reported[9]. The second comprises 15 new cases selected in a fashion to satisfy two principal aspects following our first report: i.e. the factors of mobility of the patient and duration of the anti-Parkinsonian action of the drugs. All patients in the second series were hospitalised, and all were deprived of drugs for at least 2 weeks before the urine was collected. The subjects of the first series were mainly outpatients, some of them even working, and the treatment was stopped only 24 hours before collecting the urine.

Table 1.—Clinical state of the Parkinsonism patients

	1st series	2nd series
Outpatients at work	4	0
Outpatients at home	4	0
Hospitalised but mobile	2	12
Hospitalised in bed	6	3
Total	16	15

*In the series reported in Science[7] one case has been withdrawn. After several months treatment the patient died in another hospital. An autopsy revealed that it was a case of Jakob–Creutzfeldt syndrome, although the clinical picture showed tremor and rigidity.

Table 2.—Daily excretion of catecholamines

Diagnosis	Number of cases	Urine vol. (ml/ 24hrs)	Dopamine µg/24h	Dopamine mµg/ ml	Noradrenaline µg/24h	Noradrenaline mµg ml	Adrenaline µg/24h	Adrenaline mµg/ ml
Normal Parkinsonism	31	1288	303.4	262.0	41.2	34.6	18.1	15.3
a) 1st series	15	1075	241.3	228.4	36.2	37.1	14.4	15.2
Outpatients	8	1086	257.0	243.1	34.8	38.3	14.0	16.0
Hospitalised	7	1063	222.4	211.7	36.7	35.8	15.0	14.4
b) 2nd series	15	817	198.3	292.1	51.1	75.1	14.6	21.0
Outpatients	0	—	—	—	—	—	—	—
Hospitalised	15	817	198.3	292.1	51.1	75.1	14.6	21.0
c) Total Parkinsonism	30	947	219.8	260.2	43.4	56.0	14.7	18.1

Table 2 shows the average excretion of the various catecholamines which we studied. One observes that the dopamine level is considerably reduced in relation to the normal urinary excretion. This is so both in the first and second series and in both cases the difference is statistically significant ($p < 0.01$). Several factors can, of course, influence these results, among which may be mentioned: the degree of mobility of the patient, the urinary volume, the principal symptoms.

(a) The degree of mobility: this factor is to a certain extent related to the patient's age and rigidity. When one considers that the hospitalised patient is less mobile than an outpatient (who is often working) one observes in Table 2 that his urinary volume as well as his daily excretion of dopamine are clearly diminished. However, one should note that this reduction is partly due to changes in our methods that have lowered the normal during the last few months (from 316 µg/24 hours which it was previously). One also observes that the urinary concentration of noradrenaline is higher in hospitalised patients.

(b) Urinary volume: It seems that the urinary volume in Parkinsonian subjects is reduced in relation to the norm. When this factor is taken into consideration (i.e. when one calculates the concentration of the substance) one finds that the significant difference between the two groups disappears. However, one should regard these results with suspicion because they differ from those obtained by the analysis of covariance for the complete series. In effect, whilst all the excretions of dopamine are statistically reduced to the same volume (taking into account any correlation between the two variables by covariance analysis), the urinary excretion of dopamine remains reduced in relation to normal in the Parkinsonian group ($p < 0.01$). According to Snedecor[15], it is more apposite in such a study to trust in the covariance analysis, a method that takes into account all the figures and their statistical relationship, rather than the mean of concentrations which, *a priori*, presuppose that there already exists a relationship between excretion of dopamine and the urinary volume.

In summary, despite the problem of the diminished urinary volume in Parkinsonism, it can be stated that the urinary excretion of dopamine in these subjects is lower than in normal subjects.

As the mean figures for adrenaline and noradrenaline do not differ statistically from normal in Parkinsonian subjects, it is useless to carry out the covariance analysis. However, with the addition of the second series consisting entirely of hospitalised patients, it becomes evident that the urinary concentration of noradrenaline shows an increase in Parkinsonian subjects, even though the total excretion does not differ from normal. In our opinion this explains the apparent difference between the results which we obtained previously with a biological test[7] and those obtained by biochemical estimation. In effect, in our series of 23 Parkinsonian subjects at Chicago, there were 21 hospitalised patients. The test used, based on a contraction of the aorta in the rabbit (Helmer's test) measured relatively the concentration of muscle contraction substance in the urine of a Parkinsonian subject with that of a noradrenaline standard. Ten of the 23 urines showed a contraction which we called "positive" because they surpassed the maximum contraction obtained in 235 normal ones. By this same criterion, in our series at Montreal (30 patients) there are 10 patients who have a concentration of noradrenaline exceeding 70 mμg/ml, which is the highest figure obtained in our 31 normal subjects. Thus the proportions are approximately the same in the two series.

(c) Type of the disease: it is difficult to classify the different Parkinson cases. However, if one applies the strict criteria enumerated earlier on, one observed (Table 3) that there seems to exist a

67

Table 3.—Urinary excretion of catecholamines in differing types of Parkinsonism

Diagnosis	Number of cases	Urine vol. (ml/ 24hrs)	Dopamine μg/24h	mμg/ ml	Noradrenaline μg/24h	mμg/ ml	Adrenaline μg/24h	mμg/ ml
Normal	31	1288	303.4	262.0	41.2	34.6	18.1	15.3
Parkinsonism	30	947	219.8	260.2	43.4	56.0	14.7	18.1
a) Posten- cephalitic	12	904	188.4	249.4	42.5	68.7	14.0	18.1
b) Idiopathic	15	1050	256.3	266.2	47.3	53.3	15.9	17.4
c) Arterio- sclerotic	3	617	163.0	273.7	28.0	60.3	13.0	22.0

marked difference between the postencephalitic, arteriosclerotic and "idiopathic" cases. This difference is of the same order as that observed by direct estimations in the brain by Ehringer and Horny-kiewicz[11], i.e., that lowest figures are observed in the postencepha-litis group. The number of arteriosclerotic cases is too low to allow for an evaluation, especially when one takes into account that the urinary volume is greatly reduced in this group. Thus it is justified, even biochemically, to continue separating the two main groups of Parkinsonian subjects.

(d) The principal symptoms: it seems, in view of the detailed analysis of the results, compared with the clinical and objective tests, that there is no relationship between the level of dopamine excretion and tremor; a relationship, though difficult to determine, seems on the contrary to exist between the rigidity and dopamine. The most rigid patients in these series are those who have the lowest urinary dopamine level (per 24 hours) (Fig. 1). In addition, it seems that there is an inverse relationship between the total dopamine excretion level and the concentration of noradrenaline.

2. *Overdosage with Dopa*

Because of the suspected metabolic disorders in this study, we decided to study the metabolism of an oral loading dose of 200 mg l-Dopa in normal and Parkinsonian subjects. As is known, l-Dopa is the immediate precursor of dopamine *in vivo* and that it crosses the blood-brain barrier. We tried to find out whether there is any anomaly in the conversion of exogenous Dopa into dopamine or dopacetic acid (one of the principal acid metabolites of dopamine)

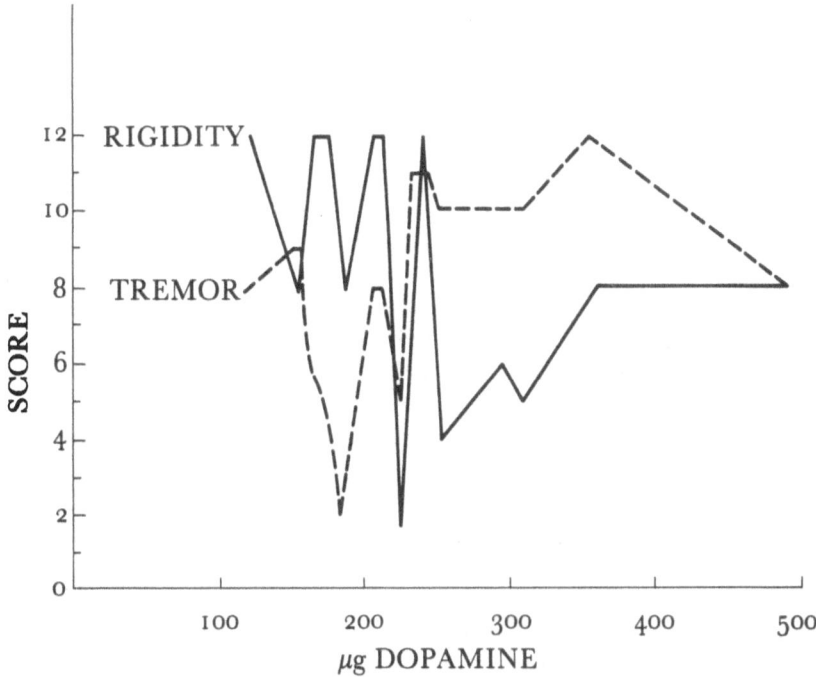

Fig. 1. — The dotted line represents the correlation between the tremor score of the 30 patients and the respective dopamine urinary excretion levels (μg/day). The solid line shows the same correlation for rigidity. It will be seen that the less the dopamine the higher the rigidity and the converse for tremor.

in our patients suffering from Parkinson's disease. The results are shown in Table 4. As can be seen, in Parkinsonian subjects the

Table 4.—Test of metabolism of exogenous Dopa

Diagnosis	Number of cases	Dopamine μg/6h	mμg/ml	Dopac μg/6h	mμg/ml	Volumes ml/6h
Control period						
Normal	6	79	23	673	190	347
Parkinsonism	8	58	31	272	150	184
After the dose						
Normal	6	5224	1090	53 729	11 210	478
Parkinsonism	8	1301	540	24 707	10 210	242

excretion of dopamine and dopac is below normal before and after the loading dose. However, in relation to volume after the loading dose, this difference disappears as regards dopac, but the concentration and the total level of dopamine remains considerably diminished when compared to normal in the Parkinsonian subjects.

Seven of the eight Parkinsonian subjects whom we studied, showed a dopamine level that was lower after the loading dose than that in the six normal subjects. Thus there is evidence that in Parkinsonian subjects the conversion of Dopa into dopamine is deficient. In order to determine this fact, it would be necessary to measure in these subjects the urinary excretion of homovanillic acid and O-methyldopamine which are also important metabolites of dopamine. Be that as it may, this conversion is due to an enzyme, the dopa-decarboxylase of which the co-enzyme is vitamin B6. It has been known for several years that this vitamin can be useful, especially against the rigidity[16,17].

Be it as it may, the difference between the urinary excretion of dopamine and dopac after the loading dose also indicates that there exists a metabolic disorder of catecholamines in Parkinson's disease. Recently Krischner[18] demonstrated that the metabolism of ^{14}C labelled exogenous noradrenaline does not differ from normal in Parkinsonian subjects. This would indicate, as is also our opinion, that the deficiency exists before this stage.

(b) *Clinical studies*

If the function of dopamine is to be a central neurotransmitter and if a disorder of the metabolism of this substance bears a relation to the Parkinson symptoms, it is logical to try to influence this symptomatology by changing the cerebral dopamine level. This can be achieved in several ways, as already demonstrated in animal experiments[19].

The following trials have been carried out in order to verify this hypothesis.

(1) by using an inhibitor of the principal enzymes of the catecholamine metabolism;
(2) by administering precursors;
(3) by combining these different methods.

1. *Use of an MAO inhibitor in Parkinson's disease*

One of the most potent MAO inhibitors, tranylcypromine ("Parnate", SKF) was used in this study in a constant dose of 10 mg three times daily. The previous treatment was continued. Thirty patients suffering from Parkinson's disease were given the treatment and the results were evaluated clinically and physically with regard to the tremor and rigidity. The results are summarised in Table 5.

Table 5.—Effect of "Parnate" in Parkinson's disease.

	Tremor		Rigidity	
	2 weeks	3 months	2 weeks	3 months
Number of cases	30	25	30	25
Initial score	244	219	224	179
Final score	138	128	171	105
Improvement %	44	41	24	41
Cases improved	24	22	20	21
Cases unchanged	5	1	7	1
Cases deteriorated	1	2	3	3
Treatment withdrawn	0	5	0	5

There was a definite and marked effect on tremor after 2 to 3 days of treatment and on rigidity after one month treatment. This effect was of the order of 40% improvement in relation to the initial state of the patient, a state was that of the optimum effect of the previous treatment.

This improvement was confirmed by a double blind test in 5 patients and by electromyographic recording in 23 patients. The details of this study have already been reported previously[21].

2. *Use of an MAO inhibitor in iatrogenic Parkinsonian syndromes*

As a control test, it seemed interesting to carry out a similar trial in 20 schizophrenics who developed a Parkinsonian syndrome after the use of phenothiazines (usually trifluoperazine). In Table 6 one observes that the results are approximately the same as those reported in the preceding paragraph, i.e. mainly improvement of the tremor and later on of the rigidity.

3. *Use of an inhibitor of the dopa-decarboxylase in Parkinson's disease*

Among the numerous inhibitors of dopa-decarboxylase, one of the most active is alpha-methyl-dopa ("Aldomet", Merck, Sharp and

Table 6.—Effect of "Parnate" in iatrogenic Parkinsonism, after 2 weeks.

	Tremor	Rigidity
Number of cases	20	20
Initial score	58	118
Final score	28	83
Improvement %	51	29
Cases improved	16	13
Cases unchanged	3	5
Cases deteriorated	1	2

addition to blocking the dopa-decarboxylase it also acts like reserpine by depleting the amine reserves, for example, the catecholamines in the brain[19], especially dopamine and serotonin. These two properties known in animals, justify a short trial of Aldomet in Parkinson's disease, in a dose of 250 mg three times daily. As could be expected, the results shown for 2 cases in Table 7 and for another 4 cases in Table 8, show that alpha-methyl-dopa rapidly aggravates

Table 7.—Alpha-methyl-dopa ("Aldomet") and reserpine in Parkinson's disease

	Rigidity score				Tremor score			
	Normal	Case 5	Case 6	Case 7	Normal	Case 5	Case 6	Case 7
a) Control period	901	489	1144	409	0	21	91	0
	1072	486	1138	331	0	16	6	0
	966	468	1166	324	0	10	99	0
Mean	979	481	1149	354	0	15	65	0
b) "Aldomet" (250 mg. t.i.d.) (or reserpine) 0.25 mg. t.i.d.) (Case 7)	950	447	1179	325	0	15	250	2
	1021	405	1172	294	0	16	90	5
	988	496	1107	291	0	21	141	10
Mean	986	449	1152	303	0	17	160	7
Percentage change	0	−6	0	—	0	−13	−170	—

the tremor and changes but little the rigidity. This effect closely resembles that which is obtained in Parkinson's disease with reserpine. An example is shown in Table 7 (case no. 7).

Table 8.—Precursors of dopamine in Parkinson's disease

Precursor	Test Other treatment	Mean number of tests	% improvement Rigidity	Tremor
l-Dopa (100 mg)		2	50	12
l-Dopa (100 mg)	Parnate	3	51	−17
l-Dopa (200 mg)		13	46	33
l-Dopa (200 mg)	"Aldomet"	2	12	−50
Tyrosine (5 g)		3	30	0
Controls				
—	"Aldomet"	4	−18	−60
—	"Kermadrin"	1	9	0
—	Placebo	3	14	0
d-Dopa (200 mg)		2	5	0
Meta-tyrosine (200 mg)		4	30	20

4. *Use of precursors of dopamine in Parkinson's disease—acute trial*

Of the immediate precursors of dopamine, we decided to study l-Dopa and tyrosine. The acute trials were carried out as follows: all previous treatment was stopped for at least 48 hours. On the morning of the trial, the patient was examined every 15 minutes for an hour by at least two examiners who evaluated the tremor and rigidity according to the scale already referred to. At 10 a.m. a dose of the compound to be studied was administered by mouth in a glass of water. Examinations were carried out every 30 minutes for 3 to 4 hours and the blood pressure was measured and the subjective sensations of the patient were noted. The doses were as follows: for l-Dopa: 100 and 200 mg, for alpha-methyl-dopa (Aldomet) 250 mg for meta-tyrosine 200 mg, "Kemadrin" (Burroughs-Wellcome) 10 mg and tyrosine 5 g; for d-Dopa 200 mg, and finally for "Parnate" 10 mg. In the majority of cases, the nature of the drug was unknown to the investigators. The results obtained are shown in Table 8. It can be seen that in all cases l-Dopa improved the rigidity, especially when it was combined with an MAO inhibitor. This improvement is of the order of 50%. It becomes manifest about 30 minutes after the ingestion and lasts 2 to 2½ hours (Fig. 2). With l-Dopa the arterial tension shows no tendency to change and the only side effect observed was slight nausea accompanied by dizziness in a patient who had already suffered from a bout of otitis. When l-Dopa was combined with an MAO inhibitor, there was sometimes a transient increase of the arterial tension

73

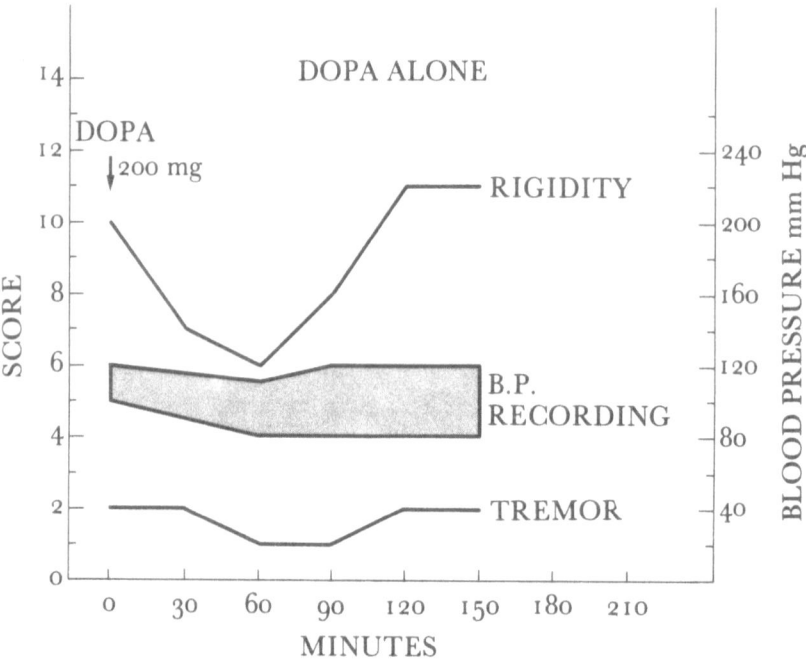

Fig. 2. – Effect of l-Dopa on rigidity, tremor and blood pressure

accompanied by an increase of tremor (Fig. 3). The tyrosine used in a dose of 5 g also improves the rigidity by about 30%. It seemed to have no effect on tremor. In order to eliminate as far as possible the placebo effect, the test was repeated on four occasions by using a capsule identical to that of l-Dopa containing no active substance and on another occasion containing 10 mg "Kemadrin". The improvement never exceeded 15% for the rigidity and there was no effect at all on the tremor.

Finally, in order to study a possible variation in the patient's state, variation independent of the drug and hour of the day, each patient was evaluated every 30 minutes for 6 hours on the eve of the test. The results shown in Table 8 take into account these slight variations which are in addition to the hourly changes.

Thus, the immediate precursors of dopamine seem to have a clear action on the rigidity. We asked ourselves the following questions: Are these effects due to the l-Dopa itself or to its conversion in dopamine? Is it a peripheral or central effect? In order to obtain a response to these questions, the following trials were carried out:

74

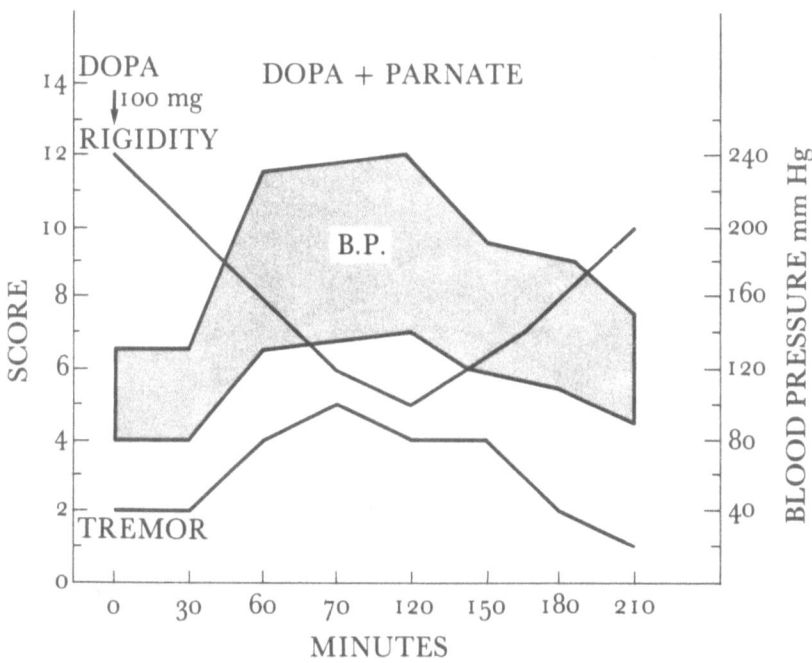

Fig. 3. — Effect of l-Dopa and "Parnate" on rigidity, tremor and blood pressure

(1) In two patients a test was carried out with l-Dopa. A few days later the patient was given 250 mg alpha-methyl-dopa ("Aldomet") and one hour later 200 mg l-Dopa and the test was repeated in the same fashion. The results obtained in the two patients were identical and is illustrated for one of them in Fig. 4. Thus, it is obvious that in the presence of an inhibitor of the dopa-decarboxylase, a loading dose of l-Dopa does not seem to improve the rigidity.

(2) We tried to increase the dopamine level by another method. To this purpose we administered 200 mg meta-tyrosine, which is known to be *in vivo* a precursor of dopamine and of meta-tyramine[23]. The results on rigidity were comparable, though inferior in equal doses to those obtained with l-Dopa, i.e. of the order of 3% (Table 8).

(3) l-Dopa is known to have a central effect and perhaps a peripheral effect. However, its non-natural isomer, the d-Dopa, is supposed to have no central effect. It is not certain that it can pass the blood-brain barrier[24]. Two patients having had a previous experience with 200 mg l-Dopa, were given a few days later an equal dose of

75

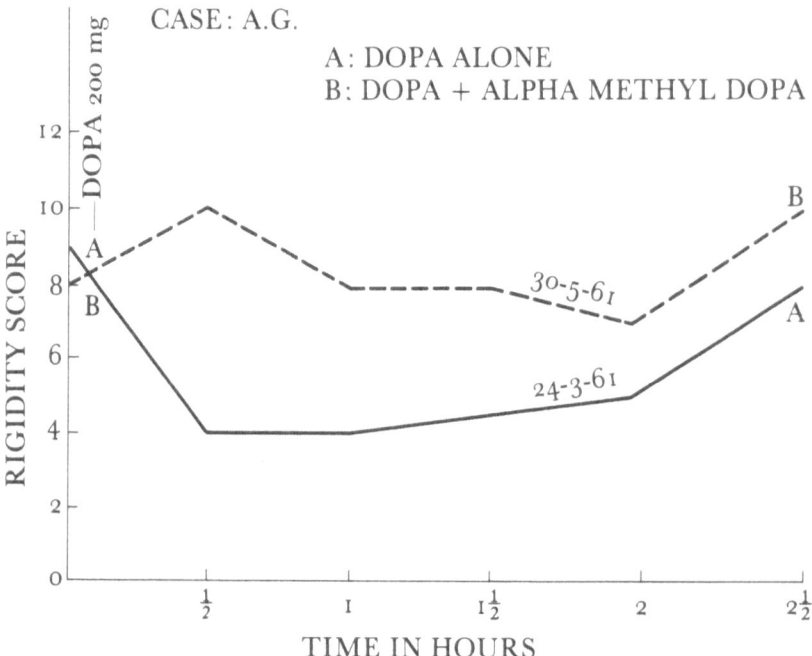

Fig. 4. — Case A. G. Comparison of the effect on rigidity of l-Dopa alone with the effect of l-Dopa and alpha methyl dopa

d-Dopa. The results obtained in these two patients were identical and are illustrated for one of them in Fig. 5. One observes that d-Dopa has no effect at all on the rigidity and tremor. Thus it appears to act better than when l-Dopa is used alone and it pro-dopamine metabolism.

5. *Use of precursors of dopamine in Parkinson's disease. Chronic trials*
Encouraged by the results of our acute tests, we tried to treat two cases of Parkinson's disease with sustained doses of l-Dopa. The results (Table 9), though preliminary, are relatively promising. In effect, it seems that l-Dopa definitely improves the rigidity. However, because of its short duration of action, it was necessary to combine it with a basic anti-Parkinsonian agent. This combination appears to act better than when l-Dopa is used alone and it produces a more marked improvement, especially where the rigidity is concerned. We hope to be able to repeat soon these trials with a

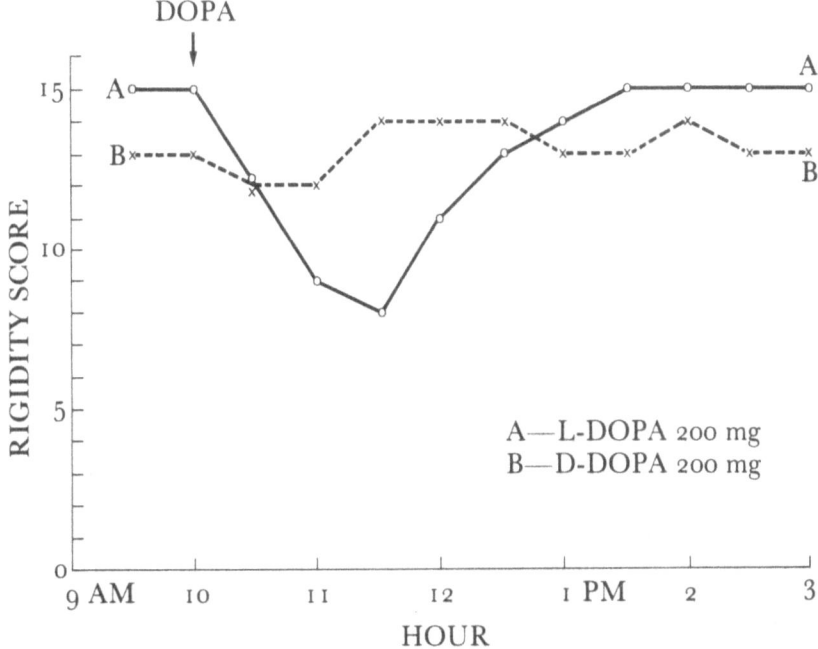

DOPA

A—L-DOPA 200 mg
B—D-DOPA 200 mg

Fig. 5. — Comparison of the effect of rigidity of l-Dopa compared with d-Dopa

Table 9.—Chronic treatment with l-Dopa in two cases of Parkinson's disease

	Experimental period	Clinical rigidity score	Performance tests. Total score
Placebo		18.7	180
l-Dopa	(100 mg × 3)	13.6	223
l-Dopa plus "Kemadrin"	(100 mg × 3) (2.5 mg × 3)	7.0	288
l-Dopa plus "Kemadrin"	(50 mg × 6) (2.5 mg × 3)	11.0	265
"Kemadrin"	(2.5 mg × 3)	5.7	326

preparation of prolonged action and with sustained doses of tyrosine.

Summary and discussion

All these tests seem to confirm our preliminary findings[7], which suggested a metabolic disorder of the catecholamines in Parkinson's

77

disease. In 1960, Ehringer and Hornykiewicz[11] demonstrated a marked reduction of the dopamine level and of noradrenaline in autopsy studies of 6 cases of Parkinson's disease. It is unlikely that this deficiency is limited to the metabolism of cerebral catecholamines, because the same substances and their enzymes are found in the whole body, especially in the liver, lungs and kidneys. If this deficiency is generalised, it is logical to study the urinary excretion of these products. This is what we have done. The results of the estimations in 30 patients who were suffering from Parkinson's disease have shown without a doubt that the excretion of dopamine in the urine is clearly diminished below the norm. This remains so even after taking into account the volumetric differences between the two groups. The type of the disease and the degree of mobility (an inverse relationship to the rigidity) seem to be important factors. In effect, the excretion of dopamine is clearly lower in postencephalitics. In addition, the rigid patients excrete less dopamine (on the whole), but have a higher urinary concentration of noradrenaline. The daily excretion of the principal metabolites of dopamine is also diminished. Our results (Table 4) show for the first time a diminution of the urinary excretion of dopac, whilst Williams *et al.*[10] had already reported that the excretion of homovanillic acid also is diminished in Parkinson's disease.

These differences of excretion are accentuated when an oral loading dose of l-Dopa is given to subjects with Parkinson's disease. It then becomes more obvious that the decarboxylation of l-Dopa in dopamine takes place with greater difficulty or at a different level than in normal subjects.

The clinical findings also seem to confirm the link between the dopamine level and certain Parkinsonian symptoms, in particular the rigidity. The use of enzyme inhibitors is non specific. At least two mechanisms of action of alpha-methyl-dopa are known and it is certain that the action can be exerted on both the catecholamine system and the metabolism of serotonin and tyramine. The same applies to the MAO inhibitors. However, it should be noted that there is an appreciable real effect and that this effect is unequal as far as rigidity and tremor are concerned. Perhaps this dichotomy is the most important factor. Alpha-methyl-dopa, the total action of which seems to be to diminish the levels of amines, aggravates the rigidity and especially the tremor. In contrast, the MAO inhibitors which increase these same amines considerably improve the tremor and to a lesser degree the rigidity.

The most convincing results are obtained with the immediate precursors of dopamine: l-Dopa, tyrosine and meta-tyrosine. In any case, these precursors, the action of which is more specific have a marked effect on the rigidity and a lesser effect on the tremor. Certain controlled trial with alpha-methyl-dopa combined with l-Dopa and with d-Dopa seem to indicate clearly that this effect on rigidity is related to a change of the cerebral dopamine level.

In conclusion, the recent clinical trials, as well as the chemical determinations in our two series of cases confirm our initial impression which permitted us to state that there is a disorder of the catecholamine metabolism in Parkinson's disease. We are increasingly more convinced that dopamine is somehow tied up with the symptoms of rigidity and that it will be necessary to discover a similar deficiency in the metabolism of other amines in order to explain the other symptoms. The important common points in the metabolism of aromatic amines are the enzymes dopa-decarboxylase and monoamine-oxidase.

References

1. Montagu, K. A.: *Catechol Compounds in Rat Tissues and in Brains of Different Animals.* Nature, *180*, 1050–1051, 1957.
2. Carlsson, A. – Lindqvist, M. – Magnusson, T. – Waldeck, B.: *On the Presence of 3-Hydroxytyramine in Brain.* Science, *127*, 471, 1958.
3. Bertler, A. – Rosengren, E.: *Occurrence and Distribution of Dopamine in Brain and Other Tissues.* Experientia (Basel), *15*, 10–11, 1959.
4. Goldstein, M. – Friedhoff, A. J. – Simmons, C.: *Metabolic Pathways of 3-Hydroxytyramine.* Biochem. and Biophys. Acta, *33*, 572–574, 1959.
5. Carlsson, A.: *The Occurrence, Distribution and Physiological Role of Catecholamines in the Nervous System.* Pharmacol. Rev., *2*, 490–494, 1959.
6. Sano, I. – Gamo, T. – Kakimoto, Y. – Taniguchi, K. – Takesada, M. – Nishinuma, K.: *Distribution of Catechol Compounds in Human Brain.* Biochem. and Biophys. Acta, *32*, 586–587, 1959.
7. Barbeau, A.: *Preliminary Observations and Abnormal Catecholamine Metabolism in Basal Ganglia Diseases.* Neurology, *10*, 446–451, 1960.
8. Barbeau, A. – Sourkes, T. L.: *Some Biochemical Aspects of Extrapyramidal Diseases.* International Symposium on the Extrapyramidal System and Neuroleptics, Montreal, Nov., 17, 1960.
9. Barbeau, A. – Murphy, G. F. – Sourkes, T. L.: *Excretion of Dopamine in Diseases of Basal Ganglia.* Science, *133*, 1706–1707, 1961.
10. Williams, C. M.: personal communication.
11. Ehringer, H. – Hornykiewicz, O.: *Verteilung von Noradrenalin und Dopamin (3-Hydroxytyramin) in Gehirn des Menschen und Ihr Verhalten bei Erkrankungen des Extrapyramidalen Systems.* Klinische Wochenschrift, *38*, 1236–1239, 1960.
12. Sourkes, T. L. – Murphy, G. F.: Methods in Medical Research, Vol. 9— Year Book Publishers, Chicago, 1961, p. 142.

13. Barbeau, A. – Duchastel, Y. – Dery, J. P. – de Groot, J. A.: *Evaluation de la Rigidité et du Tremblement dans la maladie de Parkinson.* Union Médicale du Canada. Sous presse.
14. Burns, D. B. – de Jong, J. D.: *A Preliminary Report on the Measurement of Parkinson's Disease.* Neurology, *10*, 1096–1102, 1960.
15. Snedecor, G. W.: Statistical Methods. Fourth Edition—1946. The Iowa State College Press, Ames, Iowa, 321 ff.
16. Ranco, P.: *Endorachideal Vitamin B-6 in Post-encephalitic Parkinsonism.* Rass. Stud. Psychiat., *42*, 511–519, 1953.
17. De Gouvea, L. R. L.: *Vitamin B-6 Therapy of Parkinsonism Complicating Pregnancy.* Arch. Brasil Med., *39*, 329–332, 1949.
18. Kirshner, N.: *Discussion du travail de Barbeau et Sourkes.* International Symposium on the Extrapyramidal System and Neuroleptics. Montreal, Nov. 17, 1960.
19. Sourkes, T. L.: *Formation of Dopamine* in vivo: *Relation to the Function of the Basal Ganglia.* International Symposium on the Extrapyramidal System and Neuroleptics. Montreal, Nov. 17, 1960.
20. Green, H. – Erickson, R. W.: *Effect of Trans-2-Phenylcyclopropylamine upon Norepinephrine Concentration and Monoamine Oxidase Activity of Rat Brain.* J. Pharmacol. Exp. Ther., *129*, 237–242, 1960.
21. Barbeau, A. – Duchastel, Y.: *Tranylcypromine and the Extrapyramidal Syndromes.* Can. Psych. Ass. J. In press.
22. Sourkes, T. L.: *Inhibition of Dihydroxyphenylalanine Decarboxylase by Derivatives of Phenylalanine.* Arch. Biochem. Biophys., *51*, 444, 1954.
23. Sourkes, T. L. – Murphy, G. F. – Rabinovitch, A.: *Conversion of DL-m-tyrosine to Dopamine in the Rat.* Nature, *189*, 577–578, 1961.
24. Murphy, G. F. – Sourkes, T. L.: *The Action of Anti-decarboxylases on the Conversion of 3,4-Dihydroxyphenylalanine to Dopamine* in vivo. Arch. Biochem. and Biophys., *93*, 338–343, 1961.

Part 8

Trials of Oral Therapy

*The initial trials in 1961 were followed by other studies in the early 1960s by the parenteral and the oral route (e.g. Friedhoff A. J., Hekiman L., Alpert M., and Tobach E., J. Amer. med. Ass., **184**, 285, 1963; McGeer P. L. and Zeldowicz L. R., Canad. med. Ass. J. **90**, 463, 1964: Fehling C., Acta Neurol. Scand. **42**, 7, 1966). The results of these studies were not encouraging for only a few patients showed a response and this was usually for a short duration.*

*Indeed had it not been for the fact that Cotzias and his co-workers (Cotzias G. C., Van Woert M. H. and Schiffer L. M., New Eng. Med., **276**, 374, 1967: (the paper is attached)) used gradually increasing but ultimately large oral doses (1.6 g–16 g daily) of DL-Dopa and showed that with these doses a lasting therapeutic effect could be achieved, the use of Dopa might still be only of theoretical interest. To this group should be accorded the plaudits for achieving practical therapy in Parkinsonism with Dopa. Their study involved 16 patients who were treated for periods up to almost a year. A complete or marked sustained improvement was found in 8—interestingly enough about the average rate of improvement in most subsequent large trials. Unfortunately, transient granulocytopenia was found in 4 of the patients. This was attributed to the D-form so that subsequent study and use has been of the L-form.*

Since this report in 1967 there have been many further published studies. These include uncontrolled observations, placebo-controlled and double-blind crossover within-patient trials. They now involve some 5000 patients studied for periods up to three or four years. The studies are now too extensive to give even a fraction of the individual references but there have been several recent symposia and reviews with extensive bibliographies. Among these may be quoted *Symposium on Levodopa in Parkinson's Disease—Clinical and Pharmacological Aspects* (Clin. Phar. Therap. *Vol. 12, No. 2, Part 2, pages 317–476, 1971*); *Focus on Levodopa* (Drugs **2**, *257, 1971*); *Symposium on Levodopa in Parkinson's Disease* (Neurology *Vol. 22, No. 5. Part 2, 1972*).

These extended studies show that some 5% of patients are rendered symptom free by the administration of adequate doses of levodopa and a further 60% show an improvement from their previous state on anticholinergic drugs. The recent long-term studies show that full benefit may not be achieved until treatment at maximum tolerated dosage has been continued for about six months.

Of the one third who fail to show a satisfactory response, about a quarter do not respond even on the highest tolerated dosage while the remainder probably remain at sub-therapeutic dosage levels due to intolerable side-effects. The manifestations which respond best to therapy are hypokinesia and rigidity and this is shown by improvement in a greater facility for walking, greater facial expression, improvement in dysphagia and dysarthria, improved posture and reduced drooling of saliva. On the other hand, there is a consensus of opinion that the improvement in tremor is less dramatic, less consistent and occurs later in therapy. Furthermore, some authorities insist that there is no difference between response of tremor and rigidity.

There has been no correlation of response with age or sex, but the degree of improvement shows an inverse relationship to the duration of the disease and the severity of the symptoms and signs before therapy.

There is no consistent correlation between the response and the dosage, although most patients respond best at daily dose levels of 3–6 g (average maximally effective dose about 4 g daily). There is now clear evidence that in general, patients receiving less than 3 g daily have a less satisfactory response. It is important to administer the maximum tolerated dose. Unfortunately with long-term therapy, a proportion of patients who had previously obtained substantial benefit are now showing a gradual deterioration on their motor performance. It is not clear whether this is due to the reduction of therapy or whether it has resulted from extension of the disease process.

Side-effects with levodopa therapy are troublesome. Broadly speaking they can be divided into those that occur early in therapy (and nearly all patients experience such early side-effects) and those that occur after prolonged therapy. Early side-effects usually become less troublesome if treatment can be continued although many patients find that at least some discomfort persists throughout *therapy. A dose level can however usually (in 60% patients) be found at which there is reasonable therapeutic effect without the side-effects becoming too unpleasant.*

There can scarcely be a single side-effect that has not been ascribed to levodopa but some of these are rare and some probably represent other pathological changes in the elderly patient. The main early side-effects are gastrointestinal e.g. nausea, vomiting, anorexia; cardiovascular e.g. postural hypotension, occasional arrhythmias; and behavioural, of which depression predominates. The majority of these early side-effects respond fairly rapidly to dosage reduction or cessation, and the incidence and severity of the gastrointestinal side-effects in particular can be reduced by small increments of dosage up to the maximum tolerated dose level.

Neurological side-effects tend to occur and become more troublesome at prolonged high dose levels. There are two main groups of neurological side-effects; firstly, choreoathetoid movements which usually begin in the mouth, tongue, head and neck; secondly akinesia paradoxica in which the patient suddenly and temporarily finds himself unable to move, a situation which may persist for several hours.

Another undesirable finding on long-term therapy is an alteration in hormone levels e.g. growth hormone and insulin, but clinical manifestations of these changes have not been seen so far (Yahr M. D. and Duvoisin R. C., New Eng. J. Med., **287**, *1303, 1972*).

*Reprinted from G. C. Cotzias et al., New England J. Med., **276**, No 7, 374, 1967, by kind permission of the authors and the Massachusetts Medical Society*

AROMATIC AMINO ACIDS AND MODIFICATION OF PARKINSONISM

GEORGE C. COTZIAS, MELVIN H. VAN WOERT AND
LEWIS M. SCHIFFER
UPTON, NEW YORK

The known biochemical abnormalities in Parkinson's disease consist of a decrease of melanin pigment in the substantia nigra[1,2] and a decrease of some biogenic amines in the substantia nigra and the corpus striatum[3]. These 2 defects might be interrelated, as suggested by the fact that in both melanocytes[4] and sympathetic cells[5] tyrosine is hydroxylated to dihydroxyphenylalanine, a common precursor in the synthesis of both melanin and catecholamines. Furthermore, both melanocytes and sympathetic cells originate from the neural crest[6].

It was suggested earlier[7,8] that the interrelations between melanogenesis and extrapyramidal disease might be of fundamental importance. It was noted that chronic exposure to at least 2 chemicals, manganese and phenothiazine compounds, may induce extrapyramidal manifestations. Manganese was shown to accumulate in the various melanin granules analysed[9,10], a property that is shared by phenothiazines[11]. In addition, metals such as manganese interact *in vitro* with phenothiazines to give semiquinone-free radicals, similar to those present in normal melanin[12].

In the present work an effort was made to ameliorate the known biochemical abnormalities in patients with Parkinson's disease. Initially the effect of melanocyte-stimulating hormone was investigated. This agent increases melanin deposition at least in the integumental melanocytes[13], and it was hoped that it might similarly affect the pigmented cells of the brain. Furthermore, this peptide has increased the amplitude of evoked monosynaptic potentials in the spinal cord of the cat[14]. It became apparent, however, that the Parkinsonian state was reversibly aggravated by the administration of this hormone. A serviceable working hypothesis compatible with this finding might be that the hormone was shifting dihydroxyphenylalanine (DOPA), the precursor of melanins and biogenic amines, from the brain to the integument. Therefore, it was considered desirable to investigate the therapeutic potential of DOPA, particularly since the early reports of short-lived improvement[15] were disputed by later studies[16,17,18].

Administration of higher doses than previously reported effected a striking, sustained improvement in several patients. In some of the patients depression of the circulating granulocytes and marked vacuolisation of the corresponding bone-marrow cell developed. Similar hematologic complications associated with either phenylalanine deficiency or chloramphenical toxicity have been reversed by phenylalanine[19,20]. Excesses of this amino acid have also increased the dopamine concentration in rat brain[21], and low dopamine concentrations have been linked with the pathogenesis of Parkinsonism in human beings[3]. Therefore, this amino acid was also administered. The present paper summarises these findings and discusses their relation to the therapy of Parkinsonism.

MATERIALS AND METHODS

Clinical Material

Seventeen patients with Parkinsonism were admitted to this study. All had been referred to us by their physicians, after treatment with several standard medications for relief of this disorder, including 2 who had been subjected to cryopallidectomy. All were studied as inpatients in the metabolic wards for several to many months. Some of the patients with Parkinsonism had previously participated in therapeutic studies of their disease[22]. Three without Parkinsonism were included as controls. The patients were made aware of the nature and consequences, but not of the timing, of the regimens.

Drugs and Dosages

Beta melanocyte-stimulating hormone,* with activity of 2 × $10^{(9)}$ units (Shizume-Lerner) per gram. (10 mg. per vial), was

*Kindly supplied by Armour Laboratories, Chicago, Illinois.

administered intramuscularly in 2 equal doses dissolved in 1 ml. of 16 per cent gelatin. The doses were slowly increased but did not exceed 40 mg. per day. The periods of administration were bracketed by periods of injection of the gelatin as a placebo twice daily.

D,L-phenylalanine and DL-dihydroxyphenylalanine (DOPA) were studied because of the great expense of the L-compounds. These amino acids, obtained from the Nutritional Biochemicals Corporation, were made up in pink capsules containing 100, 200 or 500 mg. The same capsules filled with lactose served as placebo. As a rule, the total number of capsules was kept constant during the evaluation of both the placebo and the amino acid.

In all studies these agents were started at a small dose that was gradually increased while the placebo was simultaneously decreased.

Laboratory Tests

A comprehensive battery of tests selected to detect evidence of drug toxicity was carried out at various intervals. The hematocrit, hemoglobin, total and differential white-cell counts, Coombs test, and platelet counts originally performed every two weeks were done twice a week after abnormalities first became apparent. The total peripheral blood granulocytes per cubic millimeter of blood were calculated by multiplication of white-cell count by the percentage of segmented and band neutrophils. Bone marrow aspirates collected in 1 per cent EDTA in saline solution were examined in 12 patients. They were immediately smeared and stained by the Wright-Giemsa method to avoid degenerative artifacts. Differential vacuole counts were made on 500 to 800 myeloid cells of 13 aspirates from 8 patients. All vacuoles were counted in thin areas of the smears and in places where there was minimal lipid deposition.

Tests of hepatic and renal function were carried out before therapy and subsequently at two-week intervals. The liver-function studies included serum protein determination with albumin-globulin ratio, serum electrophoresis, serum alkaline phosphatase, bilirubin, cholesterol, cephalin flocculation; serum glutamic oxalacetic transaminase and the bromsulfalein test. The kidney-function tests included urine-analysis, creatinine clearance, urea clearance, determination of twenty-four-hour urinary protein and occasional phosphate clearance. Weekly analyses of whole-blood manganese[23,24], serum copper and serum iron were obtained in most cases. Blood glucose, serum electrolytes, serum calcium, phosphorus, uric acid, protein-bound iodine and urinary 5-hydroxyindoleacetic acid, ferric chloride test for indoles and twenty-four-hour urinary glucose by glucose oxidase and Benedict's reaction were determined intermittently. Serum amino acid analyses before and during phenylalanine and dihydroxyphenylalanine administration are in progress.

Clinical Evaluation

Visits and periodic physical examinations were conducted twice a day in all cases. Handwriting, the number of steps required to walk 10 meters and the observed facility to sit down or stand up, to pick up an object from the floor and to draw a straight line were tested periodically. Cogwheel phenomenon, rigidity, tremor, festination, dysarthia, salivation, muscle strength and mental state were evaluated regularly, with the patients on the placebo and on the compounds tested. Cinematographic records were obtained before and during therapy in several cases.

RESULTS

Clinical

As shown in Table 1, the melanocyte-stimulating hormone was given to 6 patients. Other drugs had been withdrawn in 5 of these, and the neurological manifestations had reached a plateau. In the other patient (Case 6) this was impossible due to emergence of dysphagia. All patients initially had abdominal cramps and diarrhea, which disappeared after a few days in all but 1 (Case 4), in whom the hormone was stopped. Increased pigmentation of the skin gradually developed, most noticeably over the arms and face.

The progressive increments of the hormone induced an increase in manifestations of Parkinsonism: tremor appeared or became aggravated whereas muscular strength, posture, gait and associated movements became further impaired. Salivation emerged in 1 case, but in none was rigidity changed to an appreciable degree.

In the repeated trials of D,L-DOPA 8 (Cases 1, 6, 7, 8, 9, 10, 16 and 17) of the 16 patients showed either complete, sustained disappearance or marked amelioration of their individual manifesta-

Table 1.—Data in 20 Cases

Case No.	Age yr.	Sex	Duration of Illness yr.	Drug	Length of Therapy days	No. of Times on Placebo	Maximum Dose gm.	Maximum mg./kg.	Total Amount gm.	Improvement in Performance %
Patients with Parkinson's disease:										
1	55	F	32	Melanocyte-stimulating hormone	110	4	0.025			
				DOPA	107	5	6.0	119	282.0	>60 in performance
				Phenylalanine	50	1	12.6			
2	63	F	2	Melanocyte-stimulating hormone	68	1	0.040			
				DOPA	34	2	3.0	72	57.0	20-40 in performance
3	42	M	1½	Melanocyte-stimulating hormone	24	2	0.035			
				DOPA	108	2	10.0	93		None
				Phenylalanine	7	1	11.2			
4	57	M	3	Melanocyte-stimulating hormone	12	2	0.035			
				DOPA	44	2	10.0	128	228.0	None
5	72	F	10	Melanocyte-stimulating hormone	64	1	0.020			
6	62	M	11	Melanocyte-stimulating hormone	120	4	0.035			
				DOPA	347	7	16.0	222	3892.0	40-60
				Phenylalanine	251	2	9.0	122	1610.0	>60
7	61	M	7	DOPA	6	1	12.0			
				Phenylalanine	133	3	12.0	235	577.0	40-60
8	60	F	13	DOPA	12	2	8.0			
				Phenylalanine	163	3	12.0	195	1282.0	>60
9	60	M	8	DOPA	1	1	1.6			
10†	62	M	5½	DOPA	82	3	16.0	224	687.0	40-60
				Phenylalanine	45	2	12.0	259	330.0	20-40
11	69	F	6	DOPA	33	1	14.0	155	239.0	None
				Phenylalanine	3	3	4.0			
12	43	M	1	DOPA	10	0	8.0	122	47.0	None
13	62	M	15	DOPA	23	1	1.5	24	10.0	c
14	73	F	3	Phenylalanine	4	6	5.0			
15	59	M	1½	DOPA	38	0	9.5	125	177.4	None
16†	65	M	9	DOPA	142	2	12.0	165	1109	>60
17	54	F	6	DOPA	63	2	12.0	216	438.3	>60
Controls:										
18	80	F		DOPA	44	0	4.0	51	115.0	
19	44	F		DOPA	16	0	8.0	188	91.0	
				Phenylalanine	7	0	4.8			
20	50	M		Phenylalanine	5	0	4.0			

†Inadequate trial because of fever.   *Cryopallidectomy performed

tions of Parkinsonism. These included tremor, cogwheel phenomenon, rigidity, loss of associated movements, muscular weakness, festination, salivation and loss of facial expression. The dose required for improvement was possibly a function of the body mass (Table 1). As the dose of D,L-DOPA was gradually increased, the improvement was first noted in the rigidity, and only at higher levels was there a decrease or disappearance of tremor. The reduction in tremor was reflected in the electrocardiograms taken under identical conditions before and during therapy with D,L-DOPA. The improvement in the handwriting of one patient is shown in Figure 1. In another patient

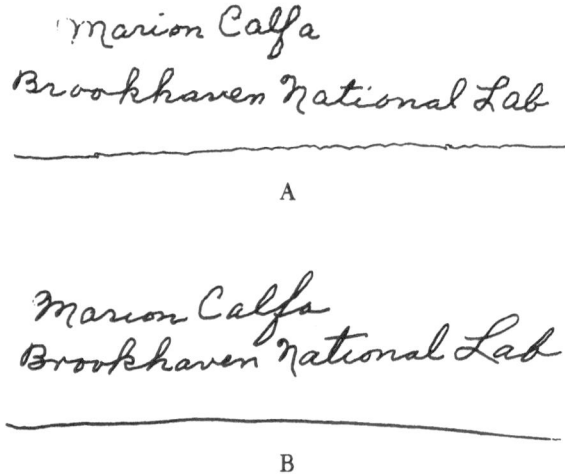

Fig. 1.—Handwriting of a patient (Case 1) before (A) and during (B) therapy with DOPA. (Note the increase in the size of the letters and the diminution of tremor.)

(Case 9), mental confusion associated with garrulity was markedly improved on this drug. This was particularly striking because every standard agent for relief of Parkinsonism tried by several physicians had either aggravated this patient's mental confusion or induced visual and auditory hallucinations. Simultaneously with motor improvement and disappearance of tremor, euphoria associated with exaggerated facial expression and gesticulation on talking developed in another patient (Case 7). These manifestations disappeared whenever the D,L-DOPA was discontinued and the full syndrome re-emerged.

In Case 6 DOPA controlled dysphagia, tremor and weakness, none of which had been significantly affected by full doses of tri-hexyphenidyl hydrochloride (Artane), ethopropazine (Parsidol), promethazine (Phenergan) or benztropine (Cogentin). Intermittent athetoid movements of the tongue were seen in this case only on DOPA. Moderate athetoid movements of all 4 extremities were exhibited by another (Case 17). Cases 10 and 16 had been subjected to cryopallidectomy elsewhere. Euphoria was not a common finding, but the sedation and "drugged" sensation associated with most therapy against Parkinson's disease was notably absent. In 2 patients (Cases 2 and 11), although sustained improvement was induced by DOPA, significant degrees of either tremor or rigidity remained. By sharp contrast, 4 (Cases 3, 4, 12 and 15) with early unilateral disease remained essentially unimproved. Case 13 became pale, apathetic and immobile on 2 trials, and DOPA was therefore not continued. In 1 (Case 14) intercurrent fever caused us to stop the drug.

In a sixty-two-year-old man with cerebral atherosclerosis and bilateral Parkinsonism transient left-sided hemiplegia developed after a total of 6.1 gm of D,L-DOPA over three days, and further therapy with this amino acid was discontinued. The control patients (Cases 18 and 19) had no discernible mental or physical consequence during administration of D,L-DOPA. Athetoid movements were observed only in patients with Parkinson's disease and only when the therapeutic effect was impressive.

Eight of the 16 patients with Parkinsonism who had received D,L-dihydroxyphenylalanine (DOPA) were subsequently given its precursor compound D,L-phenylalanine. By contrast, none of these 8 patients had any discernible improvement in their Parkinson's disease on D,L-phenylalanine, and the majority were adversely affected. Case 1 received 4 gm. of D,L-phenylalanine at the time she was enjoying marked improvement from D,L-DOPA. On this com-bination tremor, rigidity, weakness and drowsiness developed, so that the phenylalanine was discontinued. Gradual readministration of this amino acid when she was not receiving DOPA induced only a moderate aggravation of the clinical manifestations, even at a dosage level of 12.6 gm. per day. By contrast she was under sustained full control of her disease with 4.0 gm. of DOPA per day. Among the remaining 7 patients 1 (Case 11) had akinesia for the first time after receiving phenylalanine, 1 (Case 14) showed no significant changes,

91

and in the remainder minimal to moderate aggravation of the rigidity and tremor developed. Two control patients, 1 with congenital hydrocephalus (Case 19) and the other with rheumatoid arthritis (Case 20), received respectively 4.8 and 8.0 gm. of D,L-phenylalanine daily for about a week, without physical or mental changes.

Toxicologic Effects

Nausea, faintness and occasional vomiting did occur during DOPA administration, but only with increments larger than 0.5 gm. per dose. These symptoms were transitory as a rule and were not encountered with increments of less than 0.2 gm. per dose. The hematologic changes are discussed below.

Laboratory Data

The patients with Parkinsonism generally had low serum phosphorus concentrations that were unaffected by the drugs used in this study. The mean and standard deviation of 200 serum phosphorus determinations on these patients was 3.0 ± 0.5 mg. per 100 ml., with a range of 1.8 to 4.1 (normal, 3.0 to 4.5 mg. per 100 ml. by the Tausaky and Shorr method). The serum calcium, alkaline phosphatase and twenty-four-hour urinary phosphorus were all normal and unaffected by these drugs.

In 2 patients who were on long-term therapy with D,L-DOPA the blood manganese level decreased as shown in Figure 2. The lower plateau was reached in both cases after a period of DOPA administration approximating the life-span of the erythrocyte.

The remainder of the laboratory examinations were contributory only in that the urines of patients on DOPA became black on standing and showed a positive Benedict but a negative glucose oxidase reaction.

In 4 of 16 patients (Cases 1, 4, 6 and 7) granulocytopenia developed during the course of treatment with D,L-DOPA. Two episodes were rapid, and 2 gradual, the latter occurring over several months. The total granulocytes decreased to 1800 to 2300 per cubic millimeter and rose to normal, or near normal, between one week and six months after cessation of DOPA. There was no direct correlation between duration of treatment and total dose of D,L-

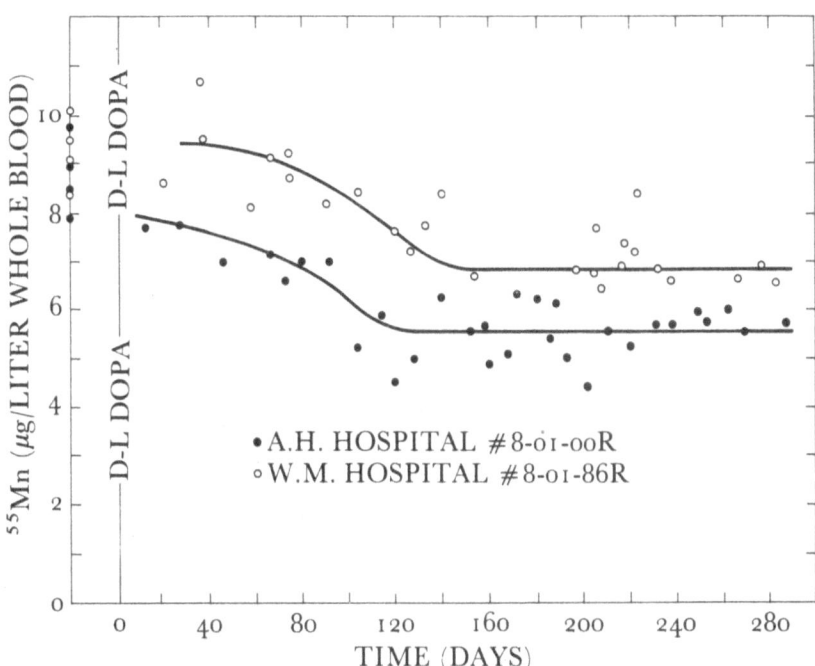

Fig. 2.—Blood manganese concentrations of 2 patients (Cases 6 and 7) as determined by neutron-activation analysis. (Note that the drop of concentration became complete after the elapse of about one hundred and thirty days.)

DOPA administered, although all cases occurred after more than 290 gm. had been consumed. There was no direct evidence of a sensitisation type of reaction. Occasional atypical lymphomonocytoid cells were seen in the peripheral blood of D,L-DOPA-treated patients, especially in those in whom granulocytopenia developed.

Quantitative and differential counting of vacuoles in cells of the myeloid series confirmed the first impressions that they were increased in numbers in bone marrows of patients treated with D,L-DOPA. The vacuoles were mostly cytoplasmic, although some overlay nuclei, and were increased in number in the more immature forms of the myeloid series (Fig. 3). The number of vacuoles per cell were also increased in blast forms, promyelocytes and myelocytes in 4 patients who were receiving, or had recently received, D,L-DOPA. Two of these patients had concomitant granulocytopenia, and 1 had previously been granulocytopenic. Only occasional vacuoles were seen in erythroid cells, and these were not quantified.

93

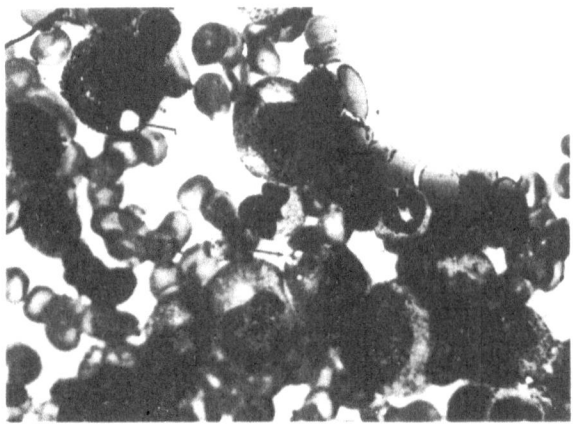

Fig. 3.—Photomicrograph of a bone-marrow smear of a patient (Case 7), showing a large vacuole in an eosinophilic myelocyte (upper left), 4 vacuoles in a myelocyte (centre) and 3 vacuoles in a metamyelocyte (lower right)

DISCUSSION

The sustained beneficial effects of DOPA observed here are in sharp contrast to some previous reports. This difference can be ascribed to the larger, sustained doses used during the present investigation. Although small doses of DOPA can reduce rigidity, the larger amounts used here are necessary to eliminate both rigidity and tremor. Some of the most striking results were obtained in patients who had advanced disease for which they had been subjected to intensive conventional medical or surgical therapy before this study. The 4 patients who did not respond significantly to the full regimen exhibited a relatively mild unilateral type of Parkinson's disease.

The mechanisms by which the effects described above were brought about remain obscure. The finding of decreased concentrations of dopamine in the brain in Parkinson's disease might have some bearing on the improvement noted in our patients. L-DOPA passes through the blood-brain barrier, leading to an increase in dopamine concentration in the brain. It is of interest that the onset of improvement when sufficient DOPA was given was rapid (within two or three hours), whereas the re-establishment of the base-line state with abrupt termination of the drug, after prolonged therapy,

94

was much longer (four to fourteen days). Long-term therapy with DOPA may well have some effect on the catecholamine storage granules that have been described[25] in certain neuron cells. If increased dopamine was the only mechanism by which improvement was brought about, one would expect effects in the same direction to follow the administration of an earlier precursor, phenylalanine. This was certainly not the case. Since the conversion of phenyl-alanine to DOPA requires hydroxylation, it is logical to suggest that defective hydroxylation of this or other aromatic amino acids might emerge as a biochemical error in this disease.

The mechanisms by which athetoid movements were induced have not been elucidated. These movements were observed only in patients with Parkinson's disease and only when the therapeutic effect of DOPA was marked.

The mode of action of melanocyte-stimulating hormone in aggravating Parkinsonism also is not clear. The stimulation of the skin melanocytes was definite, and this could have reduced DOPA available for brain metabolism. Chlorpromazine has also been reported to increase skin pigmentation[26] as well as to produce extrapyramidal symptoms[17]. Although this explanation remained speculative no further effort was made to substantiate it in view of the patients' discomfort.

The diminution of the concentration of whole-blood manganese might be worthy of comment. The time that elapsed until a new plateau was reached after administration of DOPA had approxi-mated the life-span of 1 generation of erythrocytes. This was com-patible with two earlier demonstrations: that manganese becomes incorporated in a manganoporphyrin of human erythrocytes[27], and that the exact enantiogram of Figure 2 was obtained after feeding of excessive but steady amounts of manganese as shown in Figure 2 of Cotzias *et al.*[24]. Many amino acids have significant chelating properties and are able to facilitate metal transport into cells[28]. The decrease in blood manganese could result from the redistribution of this metal by DOPA. Further investigations of this hypothesis are planned. Other essential metals have been implicated in the syndrome of Parkinsonism[29] as well as in the metabolism of some biogenic amines[30,31]. The low serum phosphorus levels encountered here, coupled with the normal calcium levels, indicate that not only manganese but also magnesium must be studied in the present context.

Administration of D,L-DOPA resulted in granulocytopenia in a sizable percentage of the patients studied. In none did infection occur, and all episodes of granulocytopenia were reversed. In 3 of the patients the drug was stopped, and in the fourth, granulocytes rose despite continued therapy. Noted in association with the granulocytopenia was extensive vacuolisation of immature cells of the myeloid series. Although there is no direct evidence linking the 2 findings it is reasonable to assume that they are related. The vacuoles seen in the bone-marrow elements are similar to those noted in the erythroid and myeloid cells of patients with phenylalanine deficiency[19] and chloramphenicol-induced erythroid suppression[20].

The sum of the evidence presented indicates that DOPA is an effective agent for certain cases of Parkinsonism and worthy of further investigation. The hematologic complications were relatively mild since they consisted of only a mild granulocytopenia and morphologic changes in the bone marrow. Still caution must be exercised in the study of D,L-DOPA. A similar long-term investigation with L-DOPA seems highly warranted as soon as it becomes economically feasible.

SUMMARY AND CONCLUSIONS

Some compounds were selected for study because of their possible effects on abnormal melanogenesis and catecholamine metabolism that occur in Parkinson's disease. These compounds included melanocyte-stimulating hormone, D,L-phenylalanine and D,L-dihydroxyphenylalanine (DOPA).

Melanocyte-stimulating hormone (20 to 40 mg.), given intramuscularly to 6 patients, resulted in an aggravation of their tremor but no significant effect on their rigidity. Oral administration of D,L-phenylalanine (1.6 to 12.6 gm.) exacerbated both tremor and rigidity in 7 out of 8 patients with Parkinson's disease.

Of the 16 patients receiving D,L-DOPA (3 to 16 gm. per day by mouth) 8 showed either complete or marked sustained improvement of several individual manifestations of Parkinsonism. Rigidity decreased or disappeared at relatively lower doses whereas only at higher levels of DOPA was there a decrease or disappearance of tremor. Two additional patients were improved but to a lesser degree by this amino acid. A significant side effect of administration of D,L-DOPA was a transient granulocytopenia encountered in 4 cases. This was associated with extensive vacuolisation of the more immature cells in the myeloid series of the bone marrow. Another side effect was the reversible induction of athetoid movements, which has been observed thus far only in patients with Parkinson's disease and only when the therapeutic effect was significant.

Although D,L-DOPA emerges as an effective therapeutic agent, the hematologic complications indicate that caution is required in further studies of this compound.

We are indebted to Mr Samuel T. Miller and Miss Judith Edwards, who performed the neutron-activation analyses for manganese, to the nurses, under the supervision of Martha Hill, R.N., for support and to Charles I. Goldman, Ph.Ch., for the expert fabrication and supply of the active chemicals and their respective placebos in the forms studied here.

References

1. Pakkenberg, H. – Brody, H.: *Number of nerve cells in* substantia nigra *in paralysis agitans.* Acta neuropathol., *5*, 320–324, 1965.
2. Duffy, P. E. – Tennyson, V. M.: *Phase and electron microscopic observations of Lewy bodies and melanin granules in* substantia nigra *and* locus caeruleus *in Parkinson's disease.* Neuropath. & Exper. Neurol., 24 398–414, 1965.
3. Hornykiewicz, O.: *Die topische Lokalisation und das Verhalten von Noradrenalin und Dopamin (3-Hydroxytyramin) in der* substantia nigra *des normalen und Parkinsonkranken Menschen.*
4. Fitzpatrick, T. B. – Seiji, M. – McGugan, A. D.: *Melanin pigmentation.* New Eng. J. Med., *265*, 328–332, 1961.
5. Udenfriend, S.: *Tyrosine hydroxylase.* Pharmacol. Rev., *18*, 43–51, 1966.
6. Boyd, J. D.: *Origin, development and distribution of chromaffin cells.* In Ciba Foundation Symposium on Adrenergic Mechanisms. Edited by J. R. Vane, G. E. W. Wolstenholme and M. O'Connor, 632 pp. London: Churchill, 1860. Pp. 63–82.
7. Cotzias, G. C. – Papavasiliou, P. S. – Van Woert, M. H. – Sakamoto, A.: *Melanogenesis and extrapyramidal diseases.* Federation Proc., *23*, 713–718, 1964.
8. Cotzias, G. C.: *Manganese, melanins and the extrapyramidal system.* J. Neurosurgery, *24*, (2), 170–175, 1966.
9. Cotzias, G. C. – Papavasiliou, P. S. – Miller, S. T.: *Manganese in melanin.* Nature (Lond.), *201*, 1228, 1964.
10. Van Woert, M. H. – Nicholson, A. R. – Cotzias, G. C.: *Functional similarities between cytoplasmic organelles of melanocytes and mitochondria of hepatocytes.* Nature (Lond.), *208*, 810, 1965.
11. Blois, M. S.: *On chlorpromazine binding in vivo.* J. Invest. Dermat., *45*, 475-481, 1965.
12. Borg. D. C. – Cortzias, G. C.: *Interaction of trace metals with phenothiazine drug derivatives.* Proc. Nat. Acad. Sc., *48*, 617–562, 1962.
13. Lerner, A. B. – Shizume, K. – Bunding, I.: *Mechanism of endocrine control of melanin pigmentation.* J. Clin. Endocrinol & Metab., *14*, 1463–1509, 1954.

14. Krivoy, W. A. – Guillemin, R.: *On possible role of β-melanocyte stimulating hormone (β-MSH) in central nervous system of mammalia: effect of β-MSH in spinal cord of cat.* Endrocrinology, *69*, 179–174, 1961.
15. Birkmayer, W. – Hornykiewicz, O.: *Der L-Dioxyphenylalanine (= L-DOPA) – Effekt beim Parkinson-syndrom des menschen Zur pathogenese und behandlung der Parkinson-Akinese.* Arch. f. Psychiat., *203*, 560–574, 1962.
16. McGeer, P. L. – Boulding, J. E. – Gibson, W. C. – Foulkes, R. G.: *Drug induced extrapyramidal reactions treatment with diphenhydramine hydrochloride and dihydroxyphenylalanine,* J.A.M.A., *177*, 665–670, 1961.
17. McGeer, P. L. – Zeldowicz, L. R.: *Administration of dihydroxyphenylalanine to Parkinsonian patients.* Canad. M. A. J., *90*, 463–466, 1964.
18. Fehling, C.: *Treatment of Parkinson's disease with L-DOPA: double blind study.* Acta neurol. Scandinav., *42*, 367–372, 1966.
19. Cockburn, F. – Sherman, J. D. – Ingall, D. – Klein, R.: *Effect of phenylalanine-deficient diet on bone marrow and amino acid metabolism.* Proc. Soc. Exper. Biol. & Med., *118*, 238–245, 1965.
20. Ingall, D. – Sherman, J. D. – Cockburn, F. – Klein, R.: *Amelioration by ingestion of phenylalanine of toxic effects of chloramphenicol on bone marrow.* New Eng. J. Med., *272*, 180–185, 1965.
21. Green, H. – Greenberg, S. M. – Erickson, R. W. – Sawyer, J. L. – Ellison, T.: *Effect of dietary phenylalanine and tryptophan upon rat brain amine levels.* J. Pharmacol. & Exper. Therap., *136*, 174–178, 1962.
22. Cotzias, G. C. – Borg, D. C. – Hughes, E. R. – Bertinchamps, A. J. – Papavasiliou, P. S.: *Phenothiazines: curative or causative in regard to Parkinsonism?* Rev. Canad. de biol., *20*, 289–294, 1961.
23. Papavasiliou, P. S. – Cotzias, G. C.: *Neutron activation analysis: determination of manganese.* J. Biol. Chem. *236*, 2365–2369, 1961.
24. Cotzias, G. C. – Miller, S. T. – Edwards, J.: *Neutron activation analysis: stability of manganese concentrations in human blood and serum.* J. Lab. & Clin. Med., *67*, 836–849, 1966.
25. Whittaker, V. P.: *Catecholamine storage particles in central nervous system.* Pharmacol. Rev., *18*, 401–412, 1966.
26. Greiner, A. C. – Berry, K.: *Skin pigmentation and corneal and lens opacities with prolonged chlorpromazine therapy.* Canad. M.A.J., *90*, 633–665, 1964.
27. Borg. D. C. – Cotzias, G. C.: *Incorporation of manganese into erythrocytes as evidence for a manganese porphyrin in man.* Nature (Lond.), *182*, 1677, 1958.
28. Neumann, P. Z. – Silverberg, M.: *Active copper transport in mammalian tissues— possible role in Wilson's disease.* Nature (Lond.), *210*, 414–416, 1966.
29. Barbeau, A. – Jasmin, G. – Duchostel, Y.: *Biochemistry of Parkinson's disease.* Neurology, *13*, 56–58, 1963.
30. Colburn, R. W. – Maas, J. W.: *Adenosine triphosphate-metal-norepinephrine ternary complexes and catecholamine binding.* Nature (Lond.), *208*, 37–41, 1965.
31. Maas, J. W. – Coburn, R. W.: *Co-ordination chemistry and membrane function with particular reference to synapse and catecholamine transport.* Nature (Lond.), *208*, 41–46, 1965.

Part 9

Relationship of Levodopa to other Forms of Therapy

It was in 1867 that Charcot (quoted in Ordenstein L., Sur la Paralysie Agitante et la Sclérase en Plaques Généralsée M.D. Thesis Paris, Martinet 1867) first advocated the use of atropine in therapy. Atropine blocks the "muscarinic" actions of acetylcholine and for almost exactly a century, atropine or synthetic drugs with muscarinic blocking action have formed the basis of conventional drug therapy of the syndrome. The estimates of the effectiveness of anticholinergic therapy vary but the general consensus is that at least 20% of patients showed a significant benefit. Indeed the only real alternative therapy until the advent of levodopa was stereotactic surgery but the long-term results were not encouraging. Thus when levodopa became available it was important to assess whether it would substitute for the anticholinergics or whether the effect of the two forms would be additive.

In many of the earlier uncontrolled observations levodopa was added to the existing treatment and these studies did not therefore really solve the problem of whether combined use offered real benefit.

One of the first definitive trials designed to study the value of combined treatment was that of Hughes and his co-workers (Hughes R. C., Polgar J. G., Weightman D. and Walton J. N., Brit. med. J. 2, 487, 1971) and this paper is reproduced here. It can be regarded as a model for clinical trials seeking to determine possible synergistic effect. The study was conducted on 34 patients stabilised on levodopa and still receiving anticholinergics. In half this number anticholinergics were withdrawn abruptly and in the remainder over a four-week period. Only 11 tolerated withdrawal of anticholinergic drugs for more than eight weeks, and these were predominantly in the slow withdrawal group. As might have been expected hypersalivation was the single feature producing the greatest problem after withdrawal, although increased slowness was a surprising complaint in view of the fact that brady-kinesia and akinesia are symptoms that respond well to levodopa.

This observation naturally raises questions of the inter-relations of abnormalities of acetylcholine and dopamine mechanisms in the genesis of Parkinsonism. It has been established that both acetylcholine and dopamine are present in high concentration in the corpus striatum where they probably act as neurotransmitters with opposing actions—dopamine inhibitory and acetylcholine excitatory. On this basis Parkinsonism with damage to the nigrostriatal pathway reduces dopaminergic function so that cholinergic dominance occurs. Hughes and his colleagues suggest that the reason why levodopa therapy is of itself inadequate may lie in the fact that the extent of striatal dopamine repletion produced is inadequate to reduce the dopaminergic/cholinergic imbalance which can therefore be further influenced by anti-cholinergic drugs.

But concomitant therapy with levodopa and anticholinergic drugs is not the only current possibility. The use of decarboxylase inhibitors is dealt with in Section 10. Simultaneous administration of pyridoxine reduces both the therapeutic effect of levodopa and certain side effects, particularly the dyskinesia (*Duvosin R. C., Yahr M. D., and Cote L. D.,* Transactions of the American Neurological Association **94**, *81, 1970*). *Pyridoxine as a co-decarboxylase probably facilitates dopamine formation preferentially outside the brain, reduces the brain effect and hence on balance is anti-therapeutic. Recently it has been discovered by chance that the anti-viral agent amantadine sometimes helps patients with Parkinsonism. The effect is often short-lived, but so far the evidence suggests that the effect is additive if levodopa is given to patients already stabilised on amantadine but not the other way round.* (*Godwin-Austen R. B., Frears C. C., Bergmann S., Parkes J. D., and Knill-Jones R. P.,* Lancet, **2**, *383, 1970, for example.*)

Reprinted from R. C. Hughes et al., Brit. Med. J., **2**, 487, 1971, by kind permission of
the authors and the British Medical Association

LEVODOPA IN PARKINSONISM: THE EFFECTS OF WITHDRAWAL OF ANTICHOLINERGIC DRUGS

R. C. HUGHES, J. G. POLGAR, D. WEIGHTMAN AND JOHN N. WALTON
THE GENERAL HOSPITAL AND THE UNIVERSITY, NEWCASTLE UPON TYNE

Summary

The results are reported of a trial in which 34 patients receiving a stable dose of levodopa for the treatment of idiopathic Parkinsonism, as well as anticholinergic drugs which they had been taking before the introduction of levodopa, underwent withdrawal of their anticholinergic remedies. Withdrawal was gradual over four weeks in 17 patients (group 1) and abrupt in the remaining 17 (group 2).

Only 11 out of 34 patients on stable levodopa therapy were able to tolerate withdrawal of anticholinergic drugs for more than eight weeks. The main reasons for the resumption of these remedies were subjective increases in slowness in 20 (59%), tremor in 15 (44%), and recurrence of hypersalivation in 5 (15%). Hypersalivation was the single feature which was most significantly and adversely influenced by anticholinergic withdrawal in patients on levodopa irrespective of whether withdrawal was sudden or gradual. It is suggested that the synergism which seems to exist between anticholinergic remedies and levodopa may be due to inhibition of dopamine inactivation by anticholinergic drugs, thus ensuring continual utilisation, or alternatively, to a primary central anticholinergic effect.

Objective and more severe subjective deterioration occurred only on sudden withdrawal. Hence we would advise that if for any reason anticholinergic drugs are to be withdrawn in patients receiving a stable dosage of levodopa this must be done slowly. Conversely it would appear from our results that the introduction of anticholinergic drugs in patients treated initially with levodopa is likely to produce additional benefit, particularly when the maximum tolerated dose of levodopa is small.

Introduction

Before treatment with levodopa became available anticholinergic drugs were the mainstay of drug treatment in Parkinsonism and produced an estimated 20% improvement (Yahr *et al.*, 1969), mainly in the features of rigidity and tremor; hypersalivation was also considerably improved in many cases. The advent of levodopa with its beneficial effects of varying degrees in all types and all aspects of Parkinsonism has raised the important question of whether anticholinergic drugs should be continued in patients receiving levodopa therapy or whether they should be given in addition when levodopa is used as the primary treatment. It is well known that rapid deterioration in the Parkinsonian state may occur when anticholinergic drugs, used as the only treatment, are withdrawn. It seemed important therefore to determine whether continued anticholinergic therapy was necessary in addition to levodopa therapy, whether any synergism existed between the two forms of treatment, and to delineate those clinical features, if any, which responded preferentially to anticholinergic drugs.

A study was therefore designed in order to analyse the effects of withdrawal of anticholinergic drugs in a group of patients receiving a stable dosage of levodopa. In view of the likelihood that sudden withdrawal would be followed by non-specific side effects patients were allocated to two groups in one of which such withdrawal was sudden and in the other gradual.

Patients and Methods

Thirty-six patients with paralysis agitans (idiopathic Parkinsonism) (20 male, 16 female) who had been receiving a constant amount of anticholinergic therapy for a number of years, and who had responded to levodopa which they had been taking in stable dosage for two months or more, were admitted to the trial. The duration of disease in these patients varied from 3 to 28 years.

Most of the patients were receiving benzhexol (Artane) or orphenadrine hydrochloride (Disipal) either alone or in combination with benztropine (Cogentin) and had been taking these drugs for at least five years. Patients were allocated to the gradual (group 1) or sudden (groups 2) withdrawal groups in such a way that the doses and combinations of anticholinergic drugs were matched as closely as possible in each group (Table 1); the groups were also matched so as to include equal numbers of patients who had undergone previous stereotaxic surgery. There were 18 patients in each group.

In group 1 anticholinergic drugs were reduced by one-quarter of the total dose per week, so that at the four-week stage these drugs had been discontinued; and in group 2 the drugs were stopped abruptly. In each group clinical assessments were carried out immediately before the trial and at two-weekly intervals thereafter for eight weeks. The patients were assessed clinically by one of two of us (R.C.H. and J.G.P.) by the methods described in a previous study (Hughes *et al.*, 1971). On this occasion, however, particular note was also made of emergent mental symptoms and autonomic release phenomena—for example, disturbances of micturition, perspiration, salivation, visual symptoms, etc. The opinions of the patients and their relatives regarding any changes were sought at each attendance and patients were told before the trial that deterioration might occur but that this was unlikely. In the event of any change occurring patients were asked if possible neither to recommence anticholinergic drugs, not to increase their dosage until they had been reassessed clinically.

Results

Two patients were eventually excluded from the study on the grounds of insufficient attendances in one case and variation of levódopa dosage in the other. Thirty-four patients therefore completed the trial period but only 16 of them were able to tolerate withdrawal and anticholinergic drugs for the whole of the eight-week trial period, and five of these 16 resumed these drugs immediately after the eight-week stage. Since then a further four patients have returned to anticholinergic therapy.

Patients' and Relatives' Assessment

Twenty-five patients felt they were worse on withdrawal of anticholinergic drugs, and their complaints, which were confirmed by

The Treatment of Parkinsonism with L-Dopa

Table I.—Prewithdrawal Dosages of Anticholinergic Drugs and Levodopa

Case No.	Benzhexol (Artane) (mg)	Orphenadrine HCl (Disipal) (mg)	Benztropine (Cogentin) (mg)	Others	Levodopa (Daily Dosage) (g)
Group 1					
1	—	200	4	—	1.2
2	—	200	2	—	1.5
3	—	—	—	Chlorphen-oxamine HCl 400 mg	4.0
4	6	—	—	Methixene HCl 15 mg	1.5
5	6	150	4	—	3.0
6	15	—	—	—	2.0
7	6	150	—	—	1.0
8	—	200	—	—	0.6
9	6	—	—	—	3.0
10	—	200	2	—	2.5
11	—	150	—	—	6.0
12	2	—	—	—	3.0
13	8	—	4	—	3.5
14	6	—	4	—	3.0
15	—	150	—	Biperiden HCl 5 mg	2.0
16	—	150	2	—	3.5
17	—	150	2	—	3.0
18*	6	—	—	—	
Group 2					
19	10	—	—	—	0.75
20	—	150	4	—	1.2
21	8	250	—	—	4.0
22	6	200	—	—	1.0
23	8	200	—	—	1.5
24	—	100	2	—	1.5
25	—	150	2	—	3.0
26	—	150	2	—	3.5
27	6	—	—	—	2.5
28	9	—	2	—	1.2
29	—	150	2	—	5.5
30	—	150	2	—	2.5
31	7.5	—	2	—	3.5
32	—	100	—	Phenglu-tarimide HCl 20 mg	4.0
33	6	—	2	—	5.0
34	—	100	2	—	4.0
35	15	150	—	—	2.0
36*	—	200	2	—	

*Withdrawn from final analysis (see text).

Table II.—Complaints of 25 patients who claimed to be worse on anticholinergic withdrawal.

	Group 1 Slow Withdrawal	Group 2 Sudden Withdrawal	Total
Increased bradykinesia	6	14	20
Increased rigidity	2	2	4
Increased tremor	8	7	15
Hypersalivation	2	3	5
Deterioration of speech	1	2	3
Dysphagia	1	1	2

their relatives, are listed in Table II. It can be seen that increasing bradykinesia, increasing tremor, or both were the commonest complaints, though in three patients gross hypersalivation was the main indication for resumption of their previous drugs. Three patients (Cases 14, 29 and 30) noted a reduction in duration of effects of individual levodopa doses from $3\frac{1}{2}$–4 hours to $2\frac{1}{2}$ hours or less; redistribution of their levodopa—that is, an increased number of doses of lesser amount—served only to reduce further the effectiveness of individual doses. This was completely reversed when anticholinergic drugs were resumed. The only factor common to these patients was that each patient was receiving benztropine (in combination with orphenadrine in two patients and benzhexol in one); other patients receiving this drug did not have similar effects. It is worthy of note, however, that two patients (Cases 24 and 28) who noted gross deterioration on withdrawal were also receiving benztropine; the deterioration in Case 28 was completely reversed by restarting benztropine alone. These findings are in accordance with the accepted fact that benztropine is the most potent anticholinergic drug in general usage. Two patients felt they were improved on withdrawal, particularly with regard to speech, and in one of these walking was said to be improved; these impressions could not be confirmed clinically.

Of the 17 patients in group 1 five said they felt no change, two felt better, and 10 felt worse. The number of patients noting deterioration is statistically significant ($P < 0.05$). Of the 17 patients in group 2, two said they felt no change, none felt better, and 15 felt worse. This again is significant ($P < 0.01$).

The Treatment of Parkinsonism with L-Dopa

Statistical Analysis

The assessment of the four main clinical features—namely, brady-kinesia, rigidity, tremor, and gait—together with the results of the four timed tests previously described (Hughes *et al.*, 1971) were analysed. The change in score from prewithdrawal to each two-weekly assessment was the measure of improvement or otherwise in the patient. Groups 1 and 2 were considered separately by these within-patient comparisons and the mean change for the group at each time interval was tested against zero (Tables III–VI).

Table III.—Group 1 patients: Walking set distance. Within-patient comparisons from prewithdrawal to two-weekly assessments

	2 weeks	4 weeks	6 weeks	8 weeks
Number of patients	17	14	12	11
Prewithdrawal mean	8.64	8.71	8.22	8.35
Mean improvement	0.89	0.94	0.77	0.86
Standard error of change	0.283	0.392	0.246	0.333
	$P < 0.01$	$P < 0.05$	$P < 0.01$	$P < 0.05$

Table IV.—Group 2 Patients: Rigidity. Within-patient comparisons from pre-withdrawal to two-weekly assessments

	2 Weeks	4 Weeks	6 Weeks	8 Weeks
Number of patients	12	9	6	4
Prewithdrawal mean	0.75	0.83	0.58	0.63
Mean deterioration	1.08	1.06	0.50	0.75
Standard error of change	0.379	0.556	0.50	0.479
	$P < 0.02$	$P > 0.05*$	$P > 0.3*$	$P > 0.02*$

*Not significant

In both groups 1 and 2 the numbers of patients able to tolerate anticholinergic withdrawal decreased progressively at each assessment interval. This was particularly so in group 2 where only four patients were able to tolerate withdrawal to the eight-week stage compared with 12 in group 1. One patient did not attend for assessment at the eight-week stage.

In group 1 there was on average a non-significant deterioration in bradykinesia, rigidity, and tremor and a non-significant improvement in gait when assessments of these features were compared with those obtained before withdrawal. Of the timed tests, repeated handgrips and rising from a chair showed on average a non-significant deterioration and restacking books a non-significant improvement. Walking a set distance, however, showed on average a significant improvement at two weeks which was maintained at the later assessments (see Table III). No reason other than anticholinergic withdrawal could be found to account for this improvement, but it should be noted that this result is in agreement with the non-significant gait improvement noted at each assessment period. It is possible that continuing improvement due to levodopa was responsible for this finding.

In group 2 patients there was on average a non-significant deterioration in all four main clinical features at two and four weeks with the exception of rigidity, which was significantly worse at two weeks (Table IV). All timed tests showed a deterioration at the two-week stage which was significant for rising from a chair ($P < 0.05$) (Table V) and higly significant for repeated handgrips ($P < 0.001$) (Table VI). At the later stages when patients unable

Table V.—Group 2 patients: Rising from a chair. Within-patient comparisons from prewithdrawal to two-weekly assessments

	2 Weeks	4 Weeks	6 Weeks	8 Weeks
Number of patients	12	9	6	4
Prewithdrawal mean	5.49	5.72	6.08	6.75
Mean change*	+8.33	+3.84	−1.12	+7.30
Standard error of change	4.197	3.812	0.931	6.921
	P <0.05	P >0.3†	P >0.3†	P >0.3†

*A positive sign indicates a deterioration
†Not significant

to tolerate withdrawal had returned to taking anticholinergic drugs, and hence could not be included in the further analysis, the changes were not significant.

When groups 1 and 2 were compared with respect to clinical features and timed tests there was a significant difference between changes noted in gait, walking a set distance, and repeated handgrips, the changes being more favourable for group 1 patients. The differences, however, were significant only at the two-week stage when there was a maximum difference between the amount of anticholinergic drugs being taken by the two groups (Tables VII–IX). After two weeks there was no significant difference between the groups in any clinical feature or timed test. For some of the timed

Table VI.—Group 2 patients: Repeated handgrips. Within-patient comparisons from prewithdrawal to two-weekly assessments

	2 Weeks	4 Weeks	6 Weeks	8 Weeks
Number of patients	12	9	6	4
Prewithdrawal mean	6.03	6.03	6.12	5.55
Mean deterioration	1.81	1.02	0.22	0.53
Standard error of change	0.406	0.552	0.549	0.384
	P < 0.001	P > 0.7*	P > 0.1*	P > 0.2*

*Not significant

Table VII.—Gait. Comparing slow withdrawal (Group 1) and sudden withdrawal (Group 2) in terms of changes from prewithdrawal to each assessment period. (Numbers of patients are shown in parentheses.)

	2 Weeks	4 Weeks	6 Weeks	8 Weeks
Mean slow withdrawal changes	−0.35 (16)	−0.21 (14)	−0.33 (12)	−0.36 (11)
Mean sudden withdrawal changes	+0.82 (11)	+0.78 (9)	−0.50 (6)	−0.50 (4)
Difference between changes	+1.17	+0.99	−0.17	−0.14
Standard error of change	0.565	0.659	0.640	0.638
	P < 0.05	P > 0.01*	P > 0.07*	P > 0.8*

*Not significant

Table VIII.—Walking set distance. Comparing slow withdrawal (Group 1) and sudden withdrawal (Group 2) in terms of changes from prewithdrawal to each assessment period. (Numbers of patients are shown in parentheses.)

	2 Weeks	4 Weeks	6 Weeks	8 Weeks
Mean slow withdrawal changes	−0.89 (17)	−0.94 (14)	−0.77 (12)	−0.86 (11)
Mean sudden withdrawal changes	+10.08 (12)	+0.30 (9)	−0.63 (6)	−0.88 (4)
Difference between changes	+10.97	+1.24	+0.14	−0.02
Standard error of change	—	—	0.448	0.682
	(Non-parametric tests)			
	P < 0.05	*	P > 0.7*	P > 0.9*

*Not significant

tests the variability of the changes experienced by the two groups was significantly different, and when this was observed the Mann-Whitney U test (instead of Student's *t* test) was used to compare the groups (Siegal, 1956) (Table VIII).

When the number of patients returning to anticholinergic therapy in group 2 were compared with those in group 1 the difference was significant at each trial interval (Table X).

Table IX.—Handgrips. Comparing slow withdrawal (Group 1) and sudden withdrawal (Group 2) in terms of changes from prewithdrawal to each assessment period. (Numbers of patients are shown in parentheses.)

	2 Weeks	4 Weeks	6 Weeks	8 Weeks
Mean slow withdrawal changes	+0.21 (17)	+0.34 (14)	+0.13 (12)	−0.91 (10)
Mean sudden withdrawal changes	+1.81 (12)	+1.02 (9)	+0.22 (6)	+0.53 (4)
Difference between changes	+1.60	+0.68	+0.09	+0.54
Standard error of change	0.564	0.861	1.032	1.257
	P <0.01	P >0.3*	P >0.9*	P >0.6*

*Not significant

Table X.—Number of patients in whom anticholinergic drugs were reintroduced

	Group 1		Group 2		
	Total in Group = 17		Total in Group = 17		
	No.	%	No.	%	
At 2 weeks	0		5	29	P = 0.044
At 4 weeks	1	6	7	41	P = 0.039
At 6 weeks	4	24	11	65	P < 0.05
At 8 weeks	5	29	13	76	P < 0.05

Mental Changes

Twenty-six patients noted no emergence of mental symptoms on withdrawal; seven had insomnia, which was associated with extremely vivid dreaming in three; and increased somnolence was noted by another patient. Four patients commented on an increase in lethargy. Depression, agitation, and confusion each occurred in two patients. Emergent mental symptoms occurred with equal frequency in groups 1 and 2 with the exception of sleep disturbance and vivid dreaming which was exclusive to group 2.

Autonomic "release" phenomena

An increase in salivation occurred in 15 patients; in most of these this relieved the levodopa-induced symptom of dryness of the mouth previously noted (Hughes *et al.*, 1971), but in five patients frank hypersalivation occurred. An increase in perspiration occurred in seven and was excessive in three. Six patients noted alteration of vision—blurring of vision occurring in three and excessive epiphora in three. Changes in bowel or bladder function occurred in seven patients, four noting relief of constipation and three complaining either of incontinence of urine or frequency and hesitancy of micturition. The urinary symptoms were relieved completely on resumption of anticholinergic therapy. When his anticholinergic drugs were withdrawn one patient developed a recurrence of ulcer dyspepsia which had been quiescent for many years.

Dyskinesia

A reduction in dyskinetic movements was noted by five patients and an increase by one patient.

Anticholinergic Dosage

Twelve of the 19 patients who restarted anticholinergic drugs before the eight-week stage found it necessary to revert to their previous dosage (100%) in order to attain their prewithdrawal status; seven, however, were able to regain this state, taking a considerably reduced dosage, the range of reduction being 23–77%.

Levodopa Dosage

The average daily dose of levodopa for the patients in the two groups was equal at 2.7 g, and in group 2 (sudden withdrawal) the dosage of levodopa being given in individual cases bore no relationship to the degree of deterioration. In group 1, however, patients who noticed no change or showed improvement on withdrawal were taking an average dose of 3.1 g compared with 2.2 g in those patients who resumed anticholinergic drugs because of deterioration.

This finding is supported by a significant association between the dosage of levodopa and the degree and direction of clinical change at the eight-week stage of slow withdrawal. The scores of the four main clinical features were combined and changes at eight weeks were plotted against the dosage of levodopa (r with 9 D.F. = −0.634 P <0.05) (Fig. 1). When changes in the combined timed

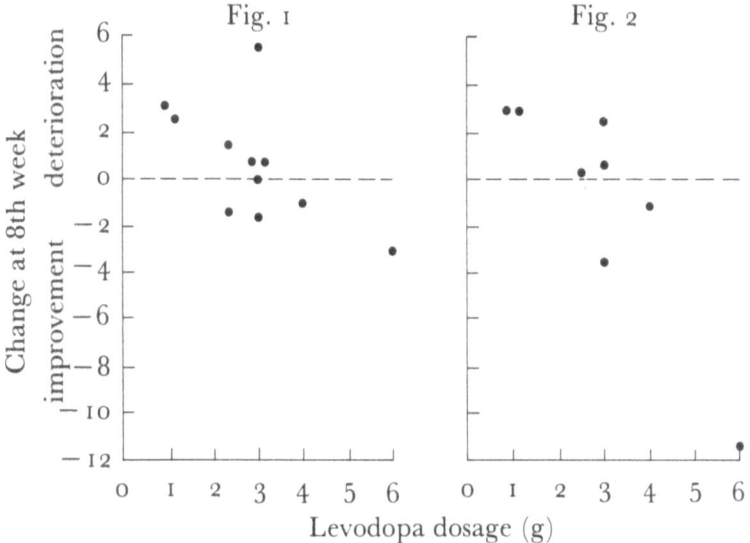

Fig. 1.—Group 1. Change in the combined scores of four clinical-features, from prewithdrawal of anticholinergic drugs to the 8th week, related to dosage of levodopa (r = −0.634, P <0.05).

Fig. 2.—Group 1. Change in the combined scores of four timed tests, from pre-withdrawal of anticholinergic drugs to the 8th week, related to dosage of levodopa (r = −0.875, P <0.01).

tests at the eight-week stage were plotted against levodopa dosage (Fig. 2) the association was significant at the 1% level. These results suggest that patients tolerating lower doses of levodopa may benefit even more than those receiving a higher dosage from the addition of anticholinergic drugs.

Previous stereotaxic surgery, either bilateral or unilateral, did not appear to influence the need to restore anticholinergic therapy, nor did the duration of the Parkinsonian syndrome.

Discussion

The fact that anticholinergic drugs could be withdrawn in only 11 of the 34 patients on stable levodopa therapy and the spectrum of symptoms which emerged during withdrawal suggest that there is a synergism between levodopa and anticholinergic drugs and that some features of Parkinsonism, especially hypersalivation, respond equally well or even preferentially to anticholinergic drugs. The increased slowness noted by 20 patients after withdrawal is surprising, since it is bradykinesia and akinesia that respond best to levodopa. However, gross deterioration in this feature was noted by only four patients. We were able to verify this clinically in one patient whose writing also showed a pronounced deterioration (Fig. 3). The other three had recommenced anticholinergic therapy,

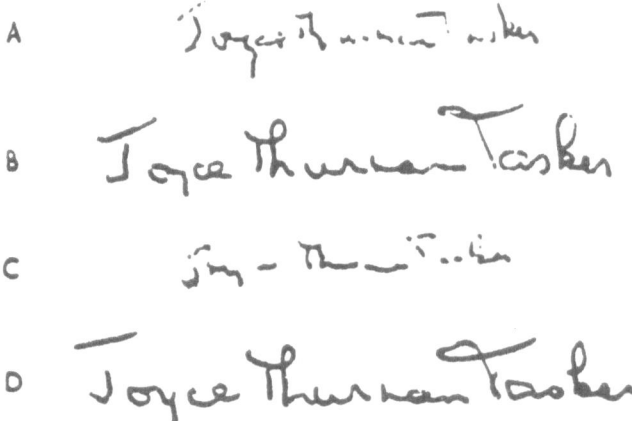

Fig. 3.—Handwriting—effect of anticholinergic withdrawal: (a) Anticholinergic drugs alone. (b) Levodopa and anticholinergic drugs (constant dose for one year. (c) One week after anticholinergic drug withdrawal (levodopa continued). (d) One week after (c)—anticholinergic drugs re-introduced.

because of gross deterioration, before they could be reassessed. The fact that only three patients were able to tolerate withdrawal beyond the eight-week stage in group 2 compared with eight in group 1 suggests that rapid withdrawal was a factor in determining these numbers, particularly since the four patients who exhibited gross deterioration on withdrawal were all in group 2. Nevertheless, even in group 1 nine patients had to return to anticholinergic therapy (which in one patient had consisted of only 2 mg of benzhexol a day) at or before the end of the trial and a further three have recommenced such treatment since the termination of the trial.

Information in the literature regarding the combined use of levodopa and anticholinergic drugs is relatively sparse, though a number of authors have commented that anticholinergic drugs were not discontinued when levodopa therapy was initiated. A possible reason why levodopa and anticholinergic drugs act synergistically is that the dopamine formed from levodopa may be inactivated by the neuronal membrane uptake system which in turn is inhibited by anticholinergic drugs as suggested by Coyle and Synder (1969). The prevention of dopamine inactivation by anticholinergic drugs gains some support from the following clinical observations noted on withdrawal of such treatment: (1) the complaints of increased slowness in 59% of patients and of increased tremor in 44%, (2) an apparent reduction in the duration of the effect of individual doses of levodopa in three patients, and (3) decrease in levodopa-induced involuntary movements in five patients by the resumption of anticholinergic drugs.

An alternative and perhaps more likely explanation for the synergism of levodopa and anticholinergic drugs is that levodopa therapy, while producing repletion of striatal dopamine, still cannot completely redress the dopaminergic/cholinergic imbalance and that a central anticholinergic effect is still required to produce a maximum therapeutic effect.

References

Coyle, J. T. – Snyder, S. H.: Science, *166*, 899, 1969.
Hughes, R. C. – Polgar, J. G. – Weightman, D. – Walton, J. N.: British Medical Journal, *1*, 7, 1971.
Siegel, S.: *In Non-parametric Statistics for the Behavioral Sciences*, p. 116, ed. S. Siegel, London, McGraw Hill, 1956.
Yahr, M. D. – Duvoisin, R. C. – Schear, M. J. – Barrett, R. E. – Hoehn, M. M.: Archives of Neurology, *21*, 343, 1969.

Part 10

Rationale and Experience of the Concomitant Administration of Decarboxylase Inhibitors and Levodopa

The effects that have followed the administration of levodopa have been attributed to its catabolism to dopamine. This occurs not only in the brain but also in peripheral tissues. This change depends on a pyridoxine-dependent enzyme usually referred to as dopa decarboxylase. This enzyme shows greater activity in animals and man in peripheral tissues (e.g. heart, liver, lung and kidney) than in the brain (mainly caudate nucleus and putamen). It is considered that brain levels following levodopa administration are lower than they would otherwise be as a result of prior peripheral levodopa metabolism and that the dopamine thus formed outside the brain tissue may account for some of the undesirable side-effects.

Thus, in theory, a peripheral decarboxylase inhibitor which did not penetrate the blood-brain barrier might permit a reduction in the levodopa dosage and the side-effects.

Reports are now available on various dopa decarboxylase inhibitors in animals and man. The first paper selected (by Pletscher A. and Bartholini G., Clin. Pharmac. Therap., **12**, *344*, *1971*) *is concerned not only with actions of one of the main compounds* (N'−(D,L-seryl)−N''−(2,3,4-tri-hydroxybenzyl) *hydrazine hydrochloride* (Ro4−4602) *in animals but also with its effects on levodopa metabolism in man. It has been chosen therefore in preference to some of the earlier papers concerned solely with animal pharma-cology (e.g. the original observation on α-methyldopa hydrazine, Udenfriend S., Zaltzman—Nuremberg P., Gordon R., and Spector S.,* Molec. Pharmacol., **2**, *95*, *1966*), *and the comparative animal study of various decarboxylase inhibitors by the two authors whose later paper is reproduced* (*i.e. Bartholini G., and Pletscher A.,* J. Pharm. Pharmac., **21**, *323, 1969*).

Their animal studies and the human biochemical studies showed that after treatment with a dopa decarboxylase inhibitor, there is improved intestinal absorption of levodopa, reduced extracerebral side-effects, enhanced selectivity of action in the brain and hence reduced levodopa requirement for therapeutic use.

Following these biochemical results it is not surprising that several clinical trials have now been undertaken to determine whether the simultaneous administration of a dopa decarboxylase inhibitor significantly improves the therapeutic response to levodopa. Among the first of these was that of Birkmayer and Mentasti in Vienna (*Birkmayer W., and Mentasti M.,* Arch. Psychiat. Bervenkr., **210**, *29, 1967*) and this was followed by several others both in Europe and North America. From these various trials that of Barbeau and his co-workers (*Barbeau A., Gillo-Joffroy, L., and Mars H.,* Clin. Pharmac. Therap., **12**, *353, 1971*) has been selected for reproduction. Although their series was smaller than for example that of Siegfried et al., (*Siegfried J., Klaiber R., Perret E. and Ziegler W. H.,* German Medical Monthly, **15**, *315, 1970*) the follow-up period was in general longer and the dose of decarboxylase inhibitor less. This minimal dose of decarboxylase inhibitor may be important, for animal experiments suggest that the present inhibitors may be toxic. It is still too early to reach a definitive answer on whether in the long-term, combined therapy is significantly better than the use of levodopa alone in experienced hands. From the studies to date, however, it does appear that there are some benefits, particularly: reduced cost and easier management from the smaller dosage; less frequent dosage; more rapid achievement of and less oscillation of therapeutic effect; fewer side-effects and possibly fewer abnormal movements. It should however be noted that with combined therapy these side-effects occurred earlier and persisted for a longer period after dosage reduction.

Reprinted from A. Pletscher and G. Bartholini, Clin. Pharmacol. Ther., **12**, *No 2, 344, 1971, by kind permission of the authors and the C. V. Mosby Co.*

SELECTIVE RISE IN BRAIN DOPAMINE BY INHIBITION OF EXTRACEREBRAL LEVODOPA DECARBOXYLATION

ALFRED PLETSCHER AND GUISEPPI BARTHOLINI
HOFFMAN-LA ROCHE, BASLE

Summary

The action of Ro 4-4602 on decarboxylase of aromatic amino acids (DC) was studied in homogenates of both brain and heart to which the drug had been added and in intact rats after parenteral administration of the compound. Furthermore, investigations on the effect of Ro 4-4602 on the metabolism of levodopa were carried out in extracerebral tissues as well as in brain of intact rats. In vivo, Ro4-4602 preferentially inhibits DC of extracerebral tissues including the brain capillaries. The inhibitor markedly enhances the accumulation of levodopa in the blood. As a consequence, increased amounts of levodopa penetrate through the brain capillaries into the cerebral parenchyma where decarboxylation to dopamine occurs. The newly formed amine is preferentially localised in the extrapyramidal brain centres. Concomitantly, the endogenous 5-hydroxytryptamine (5-HT) of the brain decreases. Potential advantages of the combination inhibitor plus levodopa over levodopa alone are: enhanced intestinal absorption of levodopa, decrease of the required levodopa dose, decrease of the peripheral side effects of levodopa, and enhanced selectivity of action of levodopa in the central nervous system.

Introduction

Inhibitors of decarboxylase of aromatic amino acids (DC) were developed about a decade ago designed to counteract arterial hypertension[15]. The most potent inhibitors, i.e. hydrazine derivatives, however, had no effect in this pathologic condition. It was soon realised that decarboxylation of 3,4-dihydroxyphenylalanine (dopa) was not a limiting step in the biosynthesis of catecholamines and therefore even a marked inhibition of DC did not diminish the formation of endogenous catecholamines in vivo. In 1966, Udenfriend and co-workers[19] noticed that a DC inhibitor, MK-485 (Fig. 1), contrary to expectations, actually enhanced the dopa-

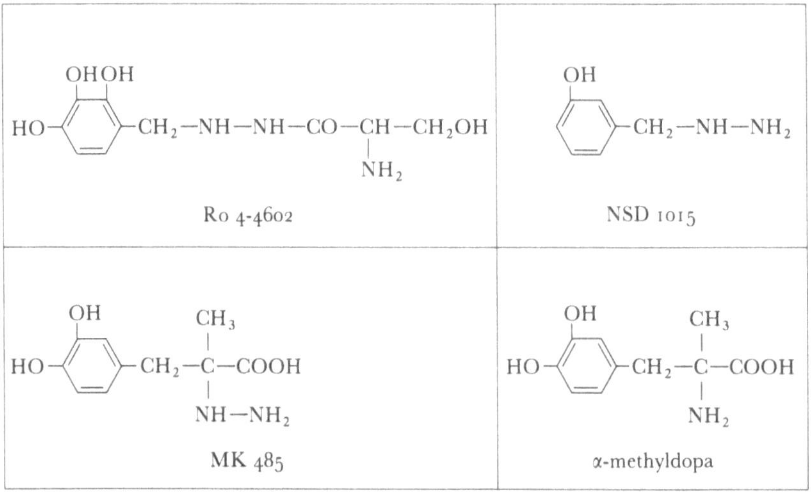

Fig. 1.—Some decarboxylase inhibitors of aromatic amino acids

induced increase of catecholamines in the brain in vivo. Furthermore, in 1967 Birkmayer[8] and Birkmayer and Mentasti[10] reported further improvement of the beneficial action of levodopa in Parkinson's disease by another DC inhibitor, Ro 4-4602. In 1967 Bartholini and associates[2] found that Ro 4-4602 enhanced the levodopa-induced increase of cerebral catecholamines; they explained these paradoxical findings as an indirect consequence of a preferential inhibition of extracerebral DC. They[2,3] also suggested combining levodopa with Ro 4-4602 in the treatment of Parkinson's disease.

Some important biochemical and histochemical findings when DC inhibitors and levodopa are combined in animals and human subjects are presented.

Chemistry and action on decarboxylase

Some DC inhibitors which have been synthesised[15] are shown in Fig. 1. With the exception of α-methyldopa, which has a relatively weak effect, they belong to the class of hydrazine or its isosters. All these compounds inhibit the transformation of dopa into dopamine in vitro and in vivo.

The addition of DC inhibitors, e.g. Ro 4-4602, to homogenates of brain and heart caused the same degree of DC inhibition in both tissues (Fig. 2). Parenteral administration of the drug to the intact

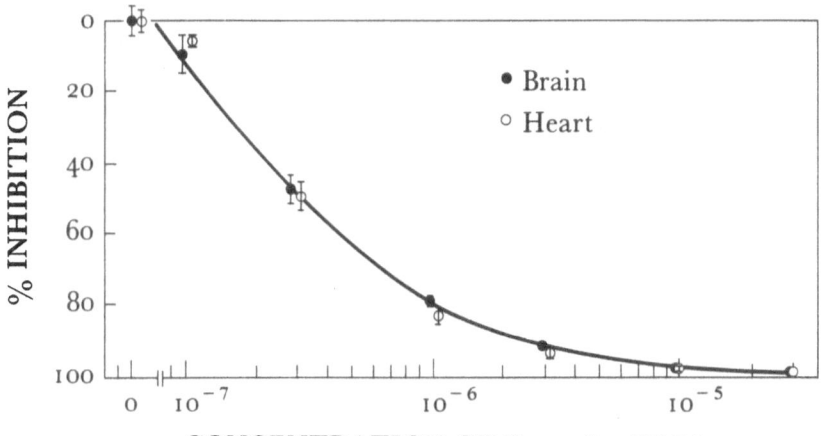

CONCENTRATION OF Ro 4-4602 IN M

Fig. 2.—Activity of decarboxylase of aromatic amino acids inhibitor by Ro 4-4602 in vitro (rats). Total homogenates (2 ml.) were incubated for one hour with 3μg of ³H-DL-dopa. The points represent averages of 4 to 6 determinations with standard error[2].

animal, however, inhibits DC more markedly in the heart than in the brain (Fig. 3). In rats, for instance, 50 mg. per kilogram of the drug intraperitoneally causes an almost complete inhibition in the heart but has no effect in the brain. Only doses as high as 300 mg. per kilogram of Ro 4-4602 inhibit the cerebral enzyme by more than 75 per cent[2,15].

From these findings it may be concluded that Ro 4-4602 preferentially interferes with extracerebral DC. This preference does not seem to be due to differences between the enzymes of the extracerebral organs and the brain, but rather to a poor penetration of the inhibitor into the brain.

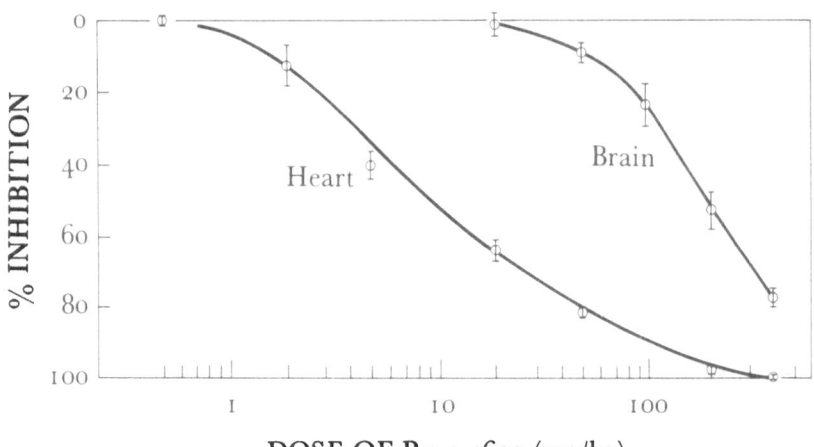

DOSE OF Ro 4-4602 (mg/kg)

Fig. 3.—Inhibition of decarboxylase of aromatic amino acids in brain and heart of rats one hour after intraperitoneal injection of Ro 4-4602. Total homogenates (2 ml.) were incubated one hour with 3μg of ^{3}H-DL-dopa. The points represent averages with standard error of 3 to 5 duplicate determinations of a pool derived from 2 to 5 animals[2].

Table I.—Distribution of the radioactivity in the different ^{14}C-catechol fractions in blood plasma and heart one hour after 16 mg. per kilogram of ^{14}C-levodopa intraperitoneally in rats with or without pretreatment with 50 mg. per kilogram of Ro 4-4602

	Blood plasma		Heart	
^{14}C-Cathechol fraction	^{14}C-dopa	Ro 4-4602 + ^{14}C-dopa	^{14}C-dopa	Ro 4-4602 + ^{14}C-dopa
Amino acids	2.99±0.05	5.70 ±0.21	1.13±0.43	4.73±0.13
Catecholamines	0.03±0.005	0.005±0.00	0.34±0.00	0.06±0.01
Phenolcarboxylic acids	2.39±0.18	0.57 ±0.02	0.76±0.23	0.26±0.02

Ro 4-4602 was administered intraperitoneally 30 minutes before ^{14}C-levodopa. The values are indicated in micromoles × 10^{-2} per milliliter of plasma or gram of heart and represent averages with standard error of 2 experiments. Each experiment was carried out with a pool of 4 to 6 animals[2].

Levodopa metabolism in animals

In the blood plasma and heart of rats, administration of relatively small doses of Ro 4-4602 (50 mg. per kilogram) markedly enhances the levodopa-induced increase of the amino acid fraction but reduces that of catecholamines and phenolcarboxylic acids, the main catecholamine metabolites (Table I)[2,3]. This action of Ro 4-4602

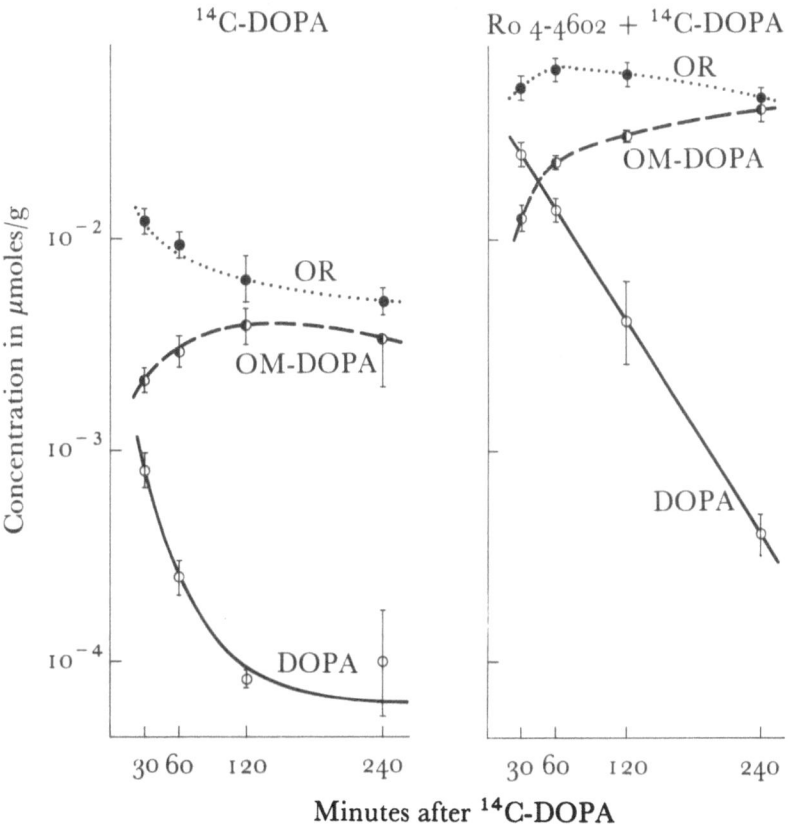

Fig. 4.—Over-all radioactivity (OR), concentration of ^{14}C-3-O-methyldopa $(OM$-$DOPA)$, and of ^{14}C-3,4-dihydroxyphenylalanine $(DOPA)$ at various time intervals after 16 mg. per kilogram of ^{14}C-levodopa intraperitoneally in brains of rats with and without pretreatment by 50 mg. per kilogram of Ro 4-4602. Ro 4-4602 was administered intraperitoneally 30 minutes before ^{14}C-levodopa. The values represent averages with standard error of 3 or 4 experiments. Each experiment was carried out with a pool of 2 brains[3].

is explained by inhibition of DC in extracerebral tissues, e.g. liver, heart, and kidney.

In the brain, Ro 4-4602 (50 mg. per kilogram) markedly enhances the levodopa-induced rise of radioactive aromatic amino acids (mainly dopa and 3-O-methyldopa), but in addition the catechola-mine fraction (mainly dopamine) is also increased. The phenol-carboxylic acids (mainly homovanillic acid and 3,4-dihydroxy-phenylacetic acid) also show a rise, but after an initial decrease (Figs. 4 and 5)[2,3].

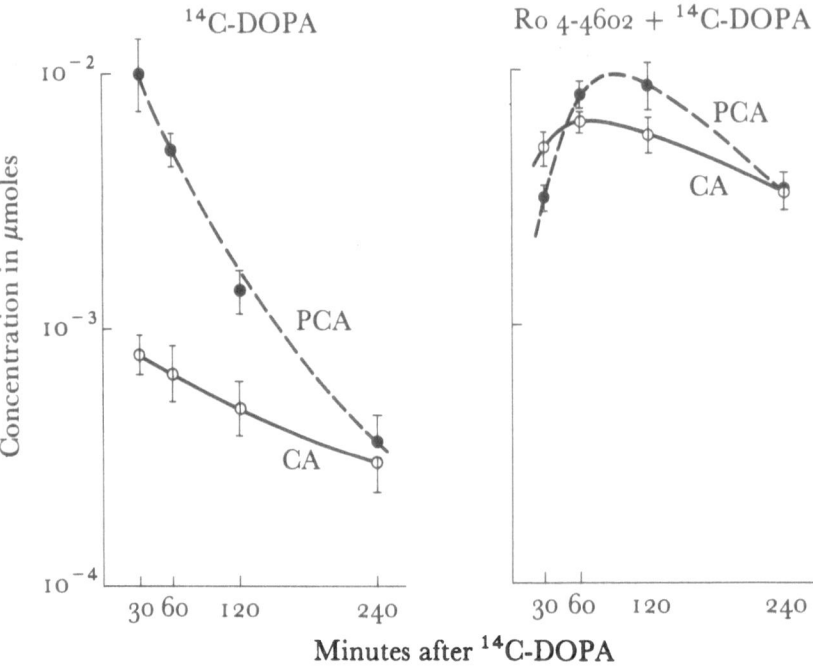

Fig. 5.—Cerebral concentration of ^{14}C-catecholamines *(CA)* and ^{14}C-phenol-carboxylic acids *(PCA)* at various time intervals after ^{14}C-levodopa intraperi-toneally in rats with and without pretreatment by 50 mg. per kilogram of Ro 4-4602. Ro 4-4602 was administered intraperitoneally 30 minutes before ^{14}C-levodopa. The values indicate averages with standard error of 3 or 4 experiments. Each experiment was carried out with a pool of 2 brains[3].

Ro 4-4602 not only enhances the levodopa-induced rise of total cerebral catecholomines, but also increases the relative amount of dopamine (as compared to norepinephrine) in the catecholamine fraction[3]. In fact, in the caudate nucleus and other brain areas, the increase of the cerebral catecholamine fraction after Ro 4-4602 plus levodopa is almost exclusively caused by dopamine (Table II).

Table II.—Enhancement of the levodopa-induced increase of catecholamines by Ro 4-4602 in the caudate nucleus of rats.

Treatment	Dopamine	Norepinephrine
Controls	6.36±0.90	0.48±0.03
Dopa	8.00±0.30	0.51±0.07
Ro 4-4602 + dopa	18.56±1.20	0.57±0.04

Levodopa, 75 mg. per kilogram, was administered intraperitoneally one hour prior to sacrifice. Ro 4-4602 (50 mg. per kilogram) was injected intraperitoneally 30 minutes prior to levodopa. The results are expressed in micrograms per gram and represent averages with standard error of 3 to 9 experiments.

It may therefore be concluded that the levodopa-induced increase of catecholamines in the brain by small doses of Ro 4-4602 is due in inhibition of extracerebral DC. As a consequence of enzyme inhibition, levodopa accumulates in the blood, and increased amounts of the amino acid penetrate the brain. This leads to an enhanced formation and accumulation of cerebral catecholamines, since the DC in the brain remains active.

Intracerebral distribution of catecholamines

Is the cerebral dopamine obtained by biochemical methods located in the parenchyma or the capillaries of the brain? By the histo-fluorimetric method of Falck and associates[12], it has been shown that in the brain a considerable part of exogenous dopa is decarboxylated and further metabolised within the capillary walls. As a consequence, dopamine, which cannot penetrate the brain parenchyma, accumulates in the capillaries, especially after inhibition of monoamine oxidase, inducing a green fluorescence of these structures [6,7,13,1]. Pretreatment with 50 mg. per kilogram of Ro 4-4602 causes the levodopa-induced green fluorescence to disappear in the capillaries, whereas in the brain parenchyma the fluorescence is enhanced (Fig. 6)[11]. This indicates that Ro 4-4602 inhibits the DC within the capillary walls, thereby protecting the dopa from being metabolised before entering the brain parenchyma. As a consequence, the majority of the amino acid can penetrate the parenchyma where, as shown biochemically, transformation into dopamine occurs since the parenchymal DC is not inhibited.

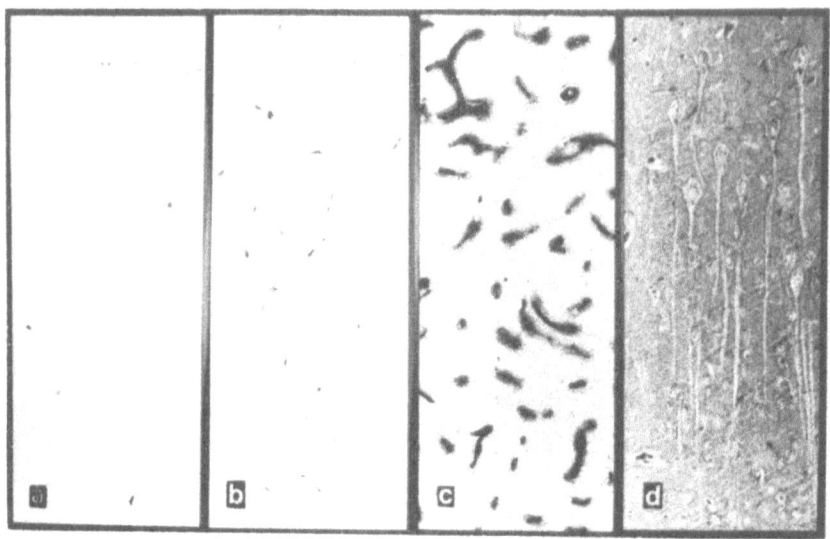

Fig. 6.—Fluorescence micrographs of the cortex of rat brain. Frontal sections. Exposure time 10 seconds. *A*, No treatment, *B*, levodopa alone, *C*, monoamine oxidase inhibator (nialamide) + levodopa, *D*, Ro 4-4602 + levodopa. Levodopa, 75 mg. per kilogram, was injected intraperitoneally either alone or 30 minutes after 50 mg. per kilogram of Ro 4-4602 intraperitoneally or 120 minutes after 259 mg. per kilogram of nialamide intraperitoneally. Sacrifice one hour after levodopa[11].

After pretreatment with Ro 4-4602, the cerebral catecholamines derived from exogenous levodopa are more specifically localised in the extrapyramidal brain centres. Thus, in animals given 50 mg. per kilogram of Ro 4-4602 plus 5 mg. per kilogram of dopa, the relative increase of catecholamines (as compared to animals treated with levodopa alone) is more pronounced in the caudate nucleus (about thirtyfold) than in other brain parts (e.g. about sevenfold in the cerebellum) (Fig. 7).

These findings indicate that Ro 4-4602 facilitates the penetration of levodopa through the brain capillaries and seems to cause a more selective localisation of the newly formed dopamine in the extra-pyramidal brain centres.

Various DC inhibitors

The differential effects of various DC inhibitors on the levodopa-

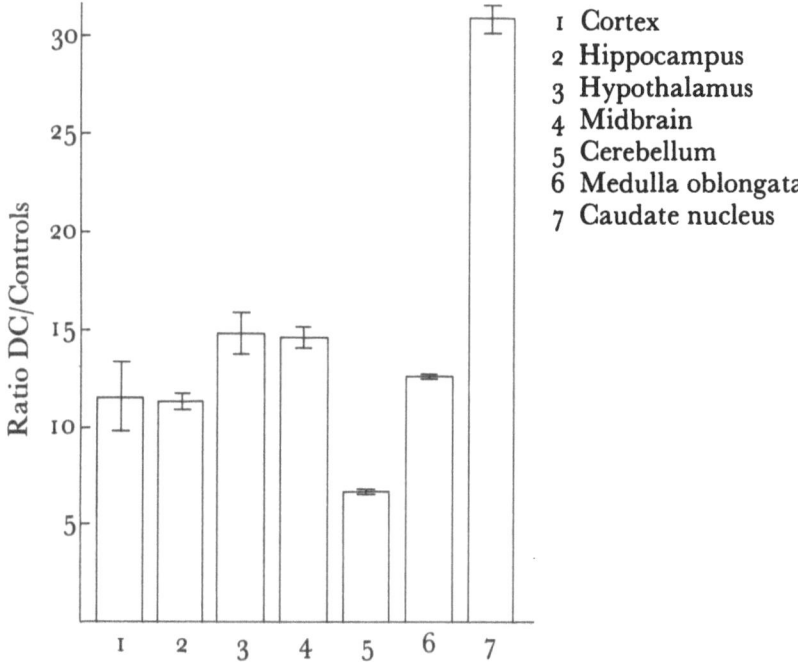

Fig. 7.—Ratio of the catecholamine increase in various brain parts. Rats were injected either with 5 mg. per kilogram of ^{14}C-levodopa intraperitoneally alone or with a combination of 50 mg. per kilogram of Ro 4-4602 intraperitoneally followed after half an hour by 5 mg. per kilogram of ^{14}C-levodopa intraperitoneally. Sacrifice 2 hours after ^{14}C-levodopa. The ordinate indicates the ratio of cerebral ^{4}C-catecholamines of animals treated with the combination (*DC*) versus those treated with dopa alone (*Controls*). The columns represent averages with standard error of 2 ratios each obtained from a pool of 6 animals treated with ^{14}C-levodopa alone and a pool of 6 animals treated with the combination ^{14}C-levodopa plus Ro 4-4602.

induced rise of catecholamines in the brain are shown in Fig. 8. α-Methyldopa has only little effect, whereas the hydrazine inhibitors—NSD 1915, Ro 4-4602, and MK-485—markedly enhance the catecholamine increase. NSD 1015 and Ro 4-4602, both rather potent compounds, reach their maximum effects with rising doses and then decrease. The diminution is probably caused by some penetration of the inhibitors into the brain parenchyma, where they interfere with the DC. Ro 4-4602 seems to penetrate the brain parenchyma less readily than does NSD 1015. Thus the effect of

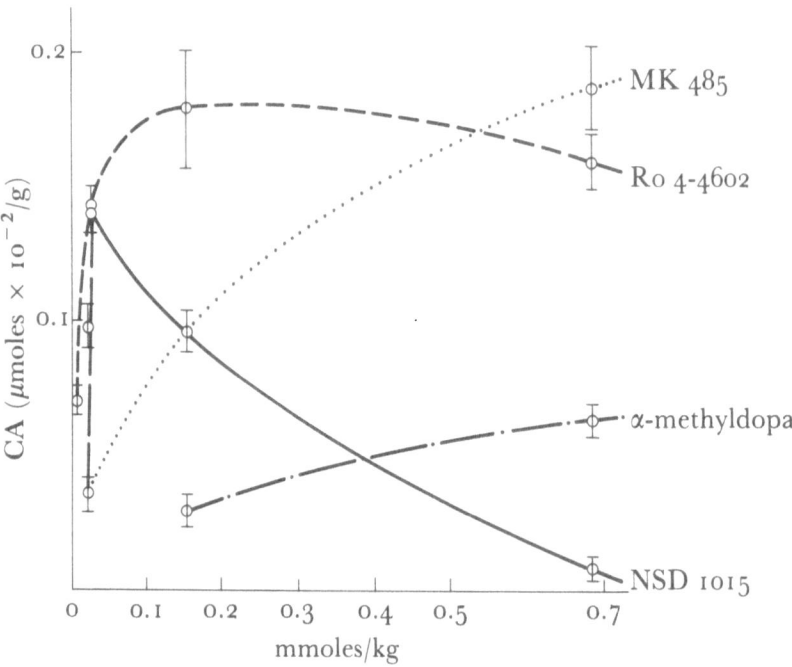

Fig. 8.—Effect of various decarboxylase inhibitors on the ^{14}C-levodopa-induced rise of ^{14}C-catecholamines in the brain of rats. The inhibitors were given 30 minutes before 3 mg. per kilogram of ^{14}C-levodopa orally; rats were killed 60 minutes after ^{14}C-levodopa. The points indicate averages with standard error of 2 to 9 experiments. The ^{14}C-catecholamine value obtained 60 minutes after ^{14}C-levodopa alone was 0.0011 ± 0.0003 μmol $\times$ 10^{-2} per gram brain[4].

Ro 4-4602 decreases only at relatively high doses of the drug, whereas NSD 1015 has a considerably narrower range of activity. MK-485 in the therapeutic dose range (1 to 10 mg. per kilogram) is less potent than the other two hydrazine inhibitors; however, it does not seem markedly to inhibit parenchymal DC of the brain at the higher doses tested[4].

Intestinal absorption of levodopa

On oral administration of levodopa alone in animals, the various catechol fractions of the brain rise to a less marked extent than they do after parenteral administration. Following pretreatment with 50 mg. per kilogram of Ro 4-4602, however, oral and parenteral administration of levodopa cause a similar increase of cerebral catecholamines[3]. This indicates that Ro 4-4602, probably due to inhibition of intestinal decarboxylation, increases absorption of levodopa. Similar conclusions have been drawn on the basis of measurements in the blood of human subjects[17].

Levodopa metabolism in human subjects

Administration orally to human subjects, Ro 4-4602 markedly enhances the levodopa-induced rise of amino acids (mainly dopa and 3-O-methyldopa) in the blood plasma and decreases that of phenolcarboxylic acids (mainly homovanillic acid and 3,4-dihydroxyphenylacetic acid)[17] (Fig. 9). This indicates that the inhibitor interferes with the extracerebral decarboxylation of levo-

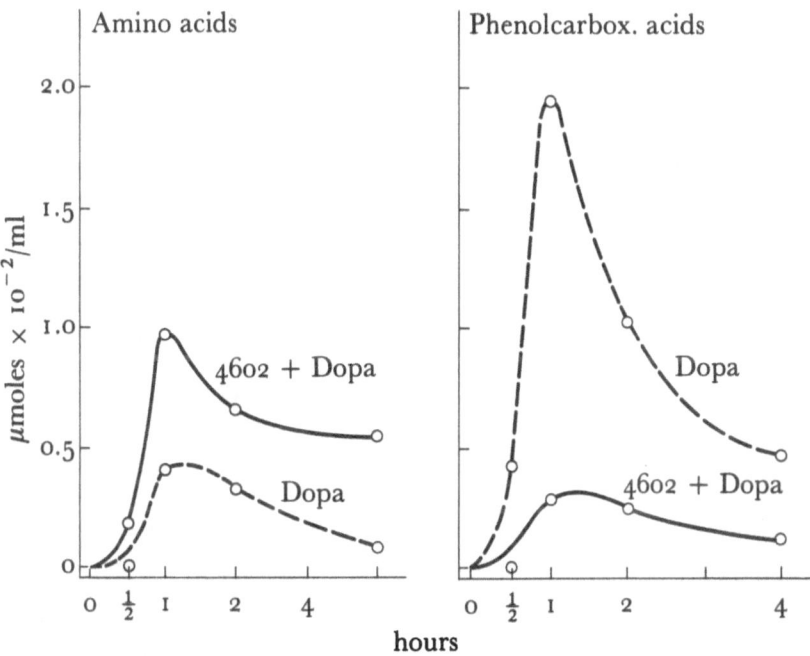

Fig. 9.—Effect of Ro 4-4602 on the ^{14}C-levodopa-induced increase of ^{14}C-amino acids and ^{14}C-catecholamines in the blood plasma of a human volunteer. In the first experiment, 3 mg. per kilogram of ^{14}C-levodopa alone was given orally. One week later, the same individual was administered both 1 mg. per kilogram of Ro 4-4602 plus 3 mg. per kilogram of ^{14}C-levodopa orally in an interval of 30 minutes.

dopa. Doses as low as 1 mg. per kilogram of Ro 4-4602 show marked activity (Fig. 9).

It can be assumed that at these low doses of Ro 4-4602 the DC activity in the human brain remains unaltered, since in animals much higher doses of the inhibitor (50 mg. per kilogram) do not interfere with the cerebral enzyme (Fig. 3).

It may therefore be concluded that, in human beings also, Ro 4-4602 probably causes a rather selective inhibition of extracerebral DC.

Metabolism of cerebral 5-hydroxytryptamine

The Ro 4-4602 plus levodopa combination decreases the endogenous 5-hydroxytryptamine (5-HT) of the rat brain. Doses as low as 50 mg. per kilogram of Ro 4-4602 plus 25 mg. per kilogram of levodopa produce a significant effect, and with higher doses of levodopa (200 mg. per kilogram) the 5-HT decreases by more than 60 per cent (Fig. 10)[5]. The diminution of cerebral 5-HT seems to be caused by several mechanisms: (1) displacement of 5-HT by dopamine, (2) competition of levodopa with the penetration of 5-HT precursors (e.g. 5-hydroxytryptophan) into the brain, (3) competitive inhibition of cerebral decarboxylation of 5-hydroxytryptophan by levodopa[5].

Conclusions

Based on experiments in animals and human subjects, the following advantages of the combination of levodopa with inhibitors of extracerebral dopa decarboxylase (DC) may be anticipated in the treatment of Parkinson's disease compared with levodopa alone.

Improved intestinal absorption of levodopa. Because of inhibition of intestinal DC, the amino acid is protected from degradation before absorption takes place.

Reduced requirements of levodopa for therapeutic use. Because extracerebral DC is inhibited, the degradation of the amino acid in peripheral organs, e.g. liver, kidney, intestine, is diminished, and a major part of levodopa is available for the brain. In addition, owing to inhibition of DC in brain capillaries, the dopa penetrating the brain parenchyma from the blood is protected from degradation in the capillary walls.

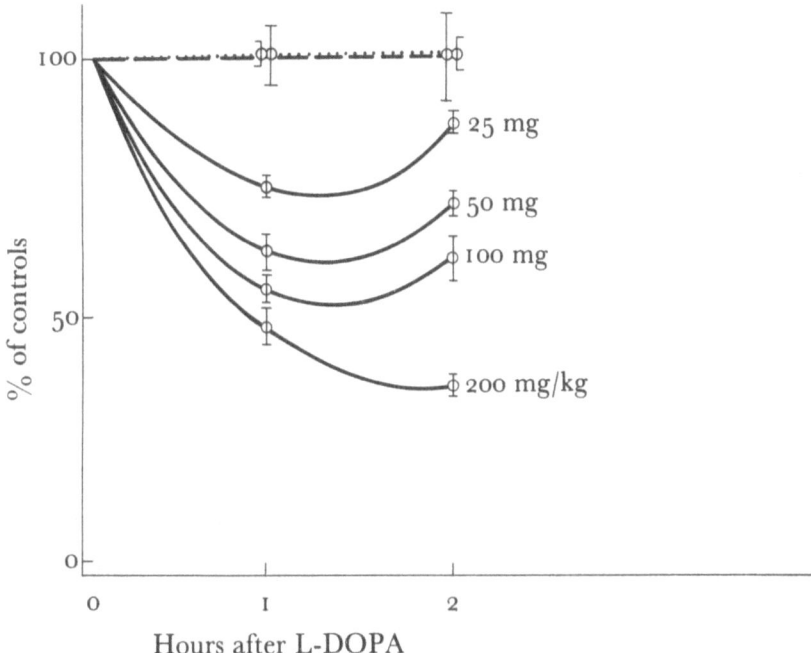

Fig. 10.—Effect of various doses of levodopa intraperitoneally (*solid lines*) on the content of endogenous 5-hydroxytryptamine (5-HT) in the brain of rats pretreated with 50 mg. per kilogram of Ro 4-4602 intraperitoneally half an hour before levodopa. The values represent averages of 3 to 4 experiments with standard error. Absolute values of cerebral 5-HT in controls: 0.35 ± 0.02 μg per gram. o . . . . . . o 200 mg. per kilogram of levodopa alone, o — — — — o 50 mg. per kilogram of Ro 4-4602 alone.

Diminution of the extracerebral side effects. Since the formation of catecholamines in the extracerebral organs is reduced, the incidence and severity of certain side effects, e.g. nausea, vomiting, arterial hyper- and hypotension, cardiac arrhythmias, may be diminished.

Enhanced selectivity of action in the brain. With the combination of Ro 4-4602 and levodopa, the newly formed dopamine is localised more selectively in the extrapyramidal brain centres, e.g. the caudate nucleus, than it is with dopa alone. The clinical action of the combination also might be more selective with regard to the extrapyramidal brain centres. Consequently, certain undesirable side effects such as psychomotor stimulation and disturbances of sleep— possibly due to catecholamines acting on other brain areas—may be relatively less pronounced.

The effect of the combination of a DC inhibitor with levodopa on endogenous brain 5-HT seems to be more pronounced than that of levodopa alone. The clinical significance of this finding is not yet clear. It remains, for instance, to be elucidated whether an interference with cerebral 5-HT metabolism influences certain symptoms of Parkinson's disease, e.g. the tremor[5].

The first clinical results of the combination Ro 4-4602 plus levodopa have been reported mainly from four centres[1,9,16,18]. The clinical findings, in some measure, bear out the experimental results. Thus, with the combination, the required levodopa dose can be reduced to about one eighth that of levodopa alone. Side effects especially those of the gastrointestinal tract and—according to some investigators—the hypotensive episodes, seem to be less frequent and less severe. The appearance of abnormal movements with the combination is less frequent according to some investigators, but according to others the incidence seems to be similar to that with levodopa alone. Serious toxicity has not been encountered, although more than 50 patients have been continuously on the combination for more than two years, and some for over three years.

Further careful clinical trials and laboratory controls should be carried out before the combination can be recommended for broad clinical use. Special attention should be given to possible long-term toxicity of the combination in human beings.

References

1. Barbeau, A. – Gillo-Joffroy, L. – Brossard, V.: *Renin, dopamine and Parkinson's disease*, in *Barbeau, A., and McDowell, F. H.*, editors: L-Dopa and Parkinsonism, Philadelphia, F. A. Davis Company. In press.
2. Bartholini, G. – Burkard, W. P. – Pletscher, A. – Bates, H. M.: *Increase of cerebral catecholamines caused by 3,4-dihydroxyphenylalanine after inhibition of peripheral decarboxylase.* Nature (Lond.), *215*, 852–853, 1967.
3. Bartholini, G. – Pletscher, A.: *Cerebral accumulation and metabolism of ^{14}C-dopa after selective inhibition of peripheral decarboxylase.* J. Pharmacol. Exp. Ther., *161*, 14–20, 1968.
4. Bartholini, G. – Pletscher, A.: *Effect of various decarboxylase inhibitors on the cerebral metabolism of dihydroxyphenylalanine.* J. Pharm. Pharmacol., *21*, 323–324, 1969.
5. Bartholini, G. – Da Prada, M. – Pletscher, A.: *Decrease of cerebral 5-hydroxytryptamine by 3,4-dihydroxyphenylalanine after inhibition of extracerebral decarboxylase.* J. Pharm. Pharmacol., *20*, 228–229, 1968.
6. Bertler, A. – Falck, B. – Owman, C. – Rosengren, E.: *The localisation of monoaminergic blood-brain barrier mechanisms.* Pharmacol. Rev., *18*, 369–385, 1966.

7. Bertler, A. – Falck, B. – Rosengren, E.: *The direct demonstration of a barrier mechanism in the brain capillaries.* Acta Pharmacol. (Kobenhavn.), *20*, 317–321, 1963.
8. Birkmayer, W.: *Die Bedeutung des Monoamin.—Metabolismus für die Pathologie des extrapyramidalen Systems.* Ars. Medici. (Liestal), *12*, 814–831, 1967.
9. Birkmayer, W.: *Experimentelle Ergebnisse über die Kombinationsbehandlung des Parkinson-Syndroms mit* L-*DOPA und einem Decarboxylasehemmer (Ro 4-4602.* Wien. Klin. Wschr., *81*, 677–679, 1969.
10. Birkmayer, W. – Mentasti, M.: *Weitere experimentelle Untersuchungen über den Catecholaminstoffwechsel bei extrapyramidalen Erkrankungen (Parkinson- und Chorea-Syndrom).* Arch. Psychiat. Nervenkr., *210*, 29–35, 1967.
11. Constantinidis, J. – Bartholini, G. – Tissot, R. – Pletscher, A.: *Accumulation of dopamine in the parenchyma after decarboxylase inhibition in the capillaries of brain.* Experientia, *24*, 130–131, 1968.
12. Falck, B. – Hillarp, N.-A. – Thieme, G. – Torp, A.: *Fluorescence of catechol amines and related compounds condensed with formaldehyde.* J. Histochem. Cytochem., *10*, 348–354, 1962.
13. Hamberger, B.: *Reserpine-resistant uptake of catecholamines in isolated tissues of the rat. A histochemical study.* Acta Physiol. Scand., *295*, Suppl., 1–56, 1967.
14. Owman, C. – Rosengren, E.: *Dopamine formation in brian capillaries—an enzymic blood-brain barrier mechanism.* J. Neurochem., *14*, 547–550, 1967.
15. Pletscher, A. – Gey, K. F. – Burkard, W. P.: *Inhibitors of monoamine oxidase and decarboxylase of aromatic amino acids,* in Eichler, O., and Farah, A., editors: Handbook of experimental pharmacology (XIX), Berlin, 1966, Springer-Verlag, pp. 593–735.
16. Siegfried, J. – Ziegler, W. H. – Regli, F. – Fischer, C. – Kaufmann, W. – Perret, E.: *Treatment of Parkinsonism with* L-*DOPA in association with decarboxylase inhibitor. First objective results.* Pharmacologia Clinica, *2*, 23–26, 1969.
17. Tissot, R. – Bartholini, G. – Pletscher, A.: *Drug-induced changes of extracerebral dopa metabolism in man.* Arch Neurol., *20*, 187–190, 1969.
18. Tissot, R. – Gaillard, J. M. – Guggisberg, M. – Gauthier, G. – De Ajuriaguerra, J.: *Therapeutique de syndrome de Parkinson par la* L-*Dopa "per os" associeé à un inhibiteur de la décarbosylase (Ro IV 46.02).* Presse Med., *77*, 619–622, 1969.
19. Udenfriend, S. – Zaltzman-Nirenberg, P. – Gordon, R. – Spector, S.: *Evaluation of the biochemical effects produced in vivo by inhibitors of the three enzymes involved in norepinephrine biosynthesis.* Molec. Pharmacol., *2*, 95–105, 1966.

*Reprinted from A. Barbeau et al., Clin. Pharmacol. Ther., **12**, No 2, 353 by kind permission of the authors and the C. V. Mosby Co.*

TREATMENT OF PARKINSON'S DISEASE WITH LEVODOPA AND RO 4-4602

ANDRÉ BARBEAU, LISE GILLO-JEFFROY AND HAROLD MARS
CLINICAL RESEARCH INSTITUTE OF MONTREAL,
HOTEL-DIEU HOSPITAL AND
UNIVERSITY OF MONTREAL

Introduction

The treatment of Parkinson's disease has known many advances in the last 15 years. Stereotaxic procedures were first introduced in 1947 by Spiegal and colleagues[41]. Modifications by Bertrand and Martinez [14] and Cooper [21] have permitted generally satisfactory results in the relief of tremor and rigidity, even if not always permanent. Bilateral symptoms of Parkinson's disease, and particularly bradykinesia, were seldom relieved and occasionally were made worse[31]. The same unresponsiveness of akinetic symptoms had been observed with the belladonna derivatives used since Charcot's[18] description in 1892 and with the synthetic anti-Parkinson drugs first introduced in 1946[25,40]. A single exception may be Schwab and co-workers[36] who recently reported favourable results with amantadine hydrochloride, a substance completely different chemically from the conventional "anticholinergic" drug.

Studies since 1959 have indicated that dopamine plays an important role in the normal physiology of the basal ganglia[27]. The observation that Parkinson's disease was partly characterised by a deficit in dopamine[11,26] led in 1960 to clinical trials with its precursor, L-dihydroxyphenylalanine (levodopa)[1,12,15]. That the symptoms of rigidity and akinesia were modified was confirmed by many[2,5], but the therapeutic value of this substance remained controversial[17] until Cotzias and associates[22,23] used larger doses of DL-dopa and later of L-dopa (levodopa). The sustained improvement obtained with a slow titration to average daily doses of 4 to 5 Gm. of levodopa has been universally confirmed[2,17,44,45].

Levodopa has produced remarkable remissions of symptoms. There is no doubt that the use of this substance offers the best currently available approach to the treatment of various signs of Parkinson's disease[2], but the high cost of the drug and problems resulting from some of the side effects[10] have justified the search for effective potentiators. Amantadine hydrochloride is partially useful in this respect[36]. In 1963, Pletscher, Gey, and Burkard[35] had prepared a new aromatic amino acid decarboxylase inhibitor: Ro 4-4602* which, in small doses, produced a selective inhibition of the peripheral enzyme, thereby permitting high levels of levodopa to reach and cross the blood-brain barrier[13]. The physiologic demonstration of this effect in man was made by Tissot and collaborators[42] and Constantinidis and associates[19]. Clinical trials with combined Ro 4-4602 and levodopa were first reported by Birkmayer and Mentasti[16] in Vienna and later confirmed by groups in Zurich[30,31,37,38,39] and Geneva[20,43]. The present paper describes our own experience with this combination over the last 14 months. In this first North American study, we were able to confirm the usefulness and advantages of this therapeutic approach to Parkinson's disease. (A preliminary report was presented at the International Congress of Neurology in September, 1969[7] and the present communication is only a progress report of the results.)

Subjects and methods

A combination of Ro 4-4602 and levodopa has been used in 23 patients for periods exceeding 3 months from March, 1969, to May, 1970. Nineteen of these suffered from Parkinson's disease of the so-called "idiopathic variety", i.e., no history of encephalitis, toxic or mechanical cause. One patient was probably postencephalitic.

The mean age of the Parkinsonian patients was 58.2 years (range 33 to 75). There were 12 men and 8 women. The average duration of the disease at onset of treatment was 8.7 years. All patients were admitted to the Hôtel-Dieu Hospital for the initial phase of evaluation and treatment and, thereafter, were seen regularly by the authors at the Parkinson Clinic of the Clinical Research Institute.

*N'-(DL-seryl)-N²-(2,3,4-trihydroxybenzyl)-hydrazine, Hoffmann-La Roche, S.A. (Basel).

The initial evaluation consisted of studies of cerebral, renal, hepatic, and blood functions. Catecholamine metabolism was also studied in each patient through the determination of urinary excretion values of dopamine, norepinephrine, epinephrine, homovanillic acid (HVA), and vanilmandelic acid (VMA). Serotonin metabolism was determined through the urinary excretion of 5-hydroxyindolacetic acid (5-HIAA) according to the method previously described[2]. In most patients the renin-aldosterone system was also investigated while the patients were on controlled intakes of sodium and in various postural conditions. These studies were done following our original observation of a defect in the renin-aldosterone system in Parkinson's disease[3,8,32].

The clinical evaluation of the patients before and during treatment consisted of a full neurological examination, a rating of their general performance according to the scale proposed by McDowell and co-workers[34] and of a battery of mechanical tests previously described to estimate rigidity and tremor[24] and to quantitate bradykinesia[28,29]. Whenever possible movie films were made of the patients before and during treatment.

At each visit to the clinic, the above clinical and mechanical evaluations were repeated. In addition, hemoglobin, hematocrit, and complete blood counts were done; glucose, blood urea nitrogen (BUN), creatinine, uric acid, alkaline phosphatase, serum glutamic oxalacetic transaminase (SGOT), lactic acid dehydrogenase (LDH), calcium, sodium, potassium, cholesterol, and total albumin were determined in the serum with the use of the SMA 12/60 automated technique. Catecholamines and 5-HIAA in the urine were determined at intervals during the treatment. Urinary calcium and phosphorus were measured by flame photometry.

The dosage of both drugs was individually adjusted and varied from subject to subject. At first we used a 1 : 1 ratio of Ro 4-4602 to levodopa as recommended by Siegfried and co-workers[39] and by Tissot and associates[43]. Because of side effects, we lowered the dose of Ro 4-4602 and now use a maximum of 200 mg. per day, the substance supplied to us in capsules containing 50 mg. of the pure powder*. Levodopa was administered in capsules of 100 mg. or 250 mg.†.

---

*We thank Dr. J. Gareau of Hoffmann-La Roche, Montreal, for supply of Ro 4-4602.

†Levodopa was purchased from Nutritional Biochemicals Corp., Cleveland, Ohio.

As recommended for the use of levodopa alone[23], it is important to reach therapeutic doses of the combination gradually and slowly. The schedule in the hospital calls for increments every third day if no side effects are encountered. We start treatment with 50 mg. of Ro 4-4602 and 100 mg. of levodopa; thereafter the increments are 50 mg. of Ro 4-4602 (not exceeding 200 mg. daily) and 100 mg. of levodopa in 1 to 4 divided doses during the day, usually at 0800, 1200, 1600, and 2000 hours. The average dose of levodopa that we have found necessary for satisfactory clinical results is 800 mg. daily, with a range of 600 to 1,500 mg. The latter dose range was used at first but is neither necessary nor recommended. Once the patients have reached a satisfactory plateau they are discharged from the hospital on a fixed dosage for the following few months. Fine adjustments of 100 mg. of levodopa are made only if necessary and as dictated by therapeutic response or side effects (chiefly involuntary movements).

Results

Clinical findings. The results obtained after a minimum of 3 months of treatment with the combination Ro 4-4602 and levodopa are summarised in Table I. As can be seen, 75 per cent of patients had more

Table I.—Results of combined therapy: Ro 4-4602, mean 200 mg. per day, and levodopa, mean 800 mg. per day.

Range of objective functional improvement (%)	Number of cases (Total N = 20)	Per cent
80–100 (very good)	9	45
50– 79 (good)	6	30
20– 49 (moderate)	4	20
0– 19 (poor)	1	5

than 50 per cent objective improvement by our tests and on the performance scale of McDowell and associates[34]. A further 20 per cent improved moderately in at least one objective measurement, but the functional improvement was not satisfactory. There was only one instance of failure in a patient who developed abnormal involuntary movements on only 300 mg. of levodopa and 150 mg. Ro 4-4602. The same patient was later treated with levodopa alone and again developed abnormal movements early, this time with

1.0 Gm per day. These results are almost identical with those we obtained after 3 months with an average daily dose of 4.8 Gm. of levodopa alone[33]. The comparison is illustrated in Fig. 1. As with

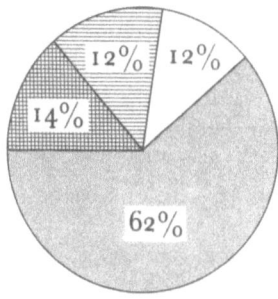 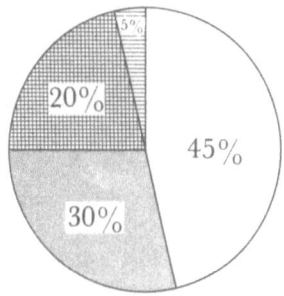

L-DOPA ALONE   L-DOPA + R04–4602
(100 *PATIENTS*)   (20 *PATIENTS*)
AVERAGE DAILY DOSE: 4.8g   AVERAGE DAILY DOSE:
     L-DOPA: 800 mg
     R04-4602 :200 mg

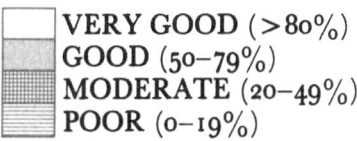

VERY GOOD (>80%)
GOOD (50–79%)
MODERATE (20–49%)
POOR (0–19%)

Fig. 1.—Comparison of results after 3 months treatment with levodopa alone and the combination of Ro 4-4602 and levodopa.

levodopa used alone[2], it may take months before the optimal level of therapy is reached. This is why we prefer to leave the patient at a less fixed daily dosage when he leaves the hospital. This dosage is usually 200 mg. of Ro 4-4602 and between 600 and 800 mg. of levodopa, depending on the individual response in the hospital.

All signs and symptoms of Parkinson's disease respond to the treatment with Ro 4-4602 plus levodopa. Bradykinesia is the first to be modified, and sometimes disappears completely, followed later by rigidity and then by tremor. We now recognise two types of tremor in Parkinson's disease. The classical—resting—slow 3 to 5 per second form, which disappears on movement, is improved in most cases after 2 to 3 months of treatment, despite an initial phase of apparent exacerbation when rigidity is gradually reduced. The second—action type—of tremor, which is occasionally seen in some patients, does not seem to respond and may even be made worse with levodopa as occurs in such entities as familial or hereditary tremor when levodopa is used.

The other beneficial effects observed with the combination Ro 4-4602 and levodopa treatment are identical with what we[2] previously described for levodopa alone.

Clinical side effects. The side effects observed when the drug was given gradually and by small increments were few, as shown in Table II. Dizziness in the early days of treatment, occasionally

Table II.—Clinical side effects of combined Ro 4-4602-levodopa therapy (20 patients, minimum 3 months of observation)

Side effects	Number	Per cent
Dizziness	7	35
Abnormal involuntary movements	6	30
Nausea and vomiting	4	20
Hypotension	3	15
Somnolence	1	5
Aggressiveness	1	5

accompanied by slight nausea, appears to be the main side effect. They were never severe enough to cause cessation of the therapeutic trial. These symptoms had completely disappeared by the time the patients left the hospital.

Abnormal involuntary movements of the type previously described[2,10] included mainly buccolingual dyskinesias and occasional dystonic or athetotic movements of the limbs. They were seen in 6 patients. It must be noted that 4 of these patients were among the first 5 treated and that they had received the combination approximately on a 1:1 ratio as recommended by Siegfried and associates[39] and Tissot and co-workers[43]. The total daily dose taken by these 4 patients averaged 1000 mg. of levodopa and 600 mg. of Ro 4-4602. Since the ratio was changed to 1:4 of Ro 4-4602 to levodopa (with a maximum daily dose of 200 mg. of Ro 4-4602), we have observed only 2 patients with temporary abnormal movements, one of whom was the hypersensitive subject described above.

We have the distinct impression that if abnormal movements are induced with the combination (especially when more than 800 mg. per day of levodopa is given), they appear sooner and take a much longer time to disappear with simple reduction of the dose as compared with our[2] previous experience with levodopa alone. In one case the movements persisted for almost 3 months after stopping both drugs. It is thus important to avoid over-treatment with levodopa with the use of fine adjustments in dosage, with immediate reduction when dystonic or athetotic movements appear.

Biochemical side effects. There have been no constant or sustained changes in any of the variables we monitored, except in the catecholamines and 5-HIAA. Rare occasional increases in BUN and/or alkaline phosphatase never lasted for more than a week and could not be correlated with clinical phenomena, dosage, or therapeutic response. We paid particular attention to liver function: over the 14 months of the study, Bromsulphalein (BSP), proteins, albumins, enzymes, and other parameters (see above), including liver scans with radioactive gold, never became abnormal. Calcium and phosphorus values, both in the blood and in the urine, remained within normal limits.

As expected, urinary dopamine and HVA values increased considerably with treatment, but we could not demonstrate valid correlations with therapeutic efficacy. There was a constant and significant decrease in the urinary excretion of 5-HIAA after 3 months of combined therapy.

Discussion

In our hands and after 14 months of observation, the combination levodopa with an inhibitor of peripheral decarboxylase (Ro 4-4602) is a useful and safe therapeutic measure in Parkinson's disease. It compares favourably with the results of levodopa therapy alone[2,33]. In fact, if long-term toxicity studies of the inhibitor at the dosage we recommend (maximum 200 mg. per day of Ro 4-4602) should prove to be acceptable, we would be of the opinion that the combination is preferable to levodopa alone. The advantages seen to date are the following: (1) lower dose of levodopa and therefore also lower cost; (2) ease of handling (With proper galenic preparations it will be possible to use only 3 or 4 capsules a day.); (3) need for fewer divided doses during the day (The inhibitor definitely prolongs the action of a single dose.); (4) fewer oscillations in daily and long-term performance (To date we have not observed the late-occurring bradykinetic and hypotonic "freezing" episodes seen after 8 to 12 months with levodopa alone[2,10]); (5) fewer side effects of nausea and hypotension; (6) possibly fewer abnormal movements, although these tend to occur earlier and may be more difficult to reduce once present; (7) earlier achievement of the therapeutic plateau, defined as a minimum of 50 per cent improvement in our functional tests.

Despite a careful surveillance of hepatic and calcium metabolism, we have not yet seen in human beings the few complications reported in animals at doses considerably higher than those used in human subjects. In personal communications, Birkmayer, Siegfried, and Tissot, whose observations now range up to 3 years, inform us they have not had difficulties of this nature in human subjects. We are nevertheless pursuing this aspect of the investigation. We have not observed any evidence of systemic lupus erythematosus in our patients under treatment.

It is not necessary to exceed the 200 mg. daily dose of Ro 4-4602 for satisfactory results. This represents a considerable reduction from the doses recommended previously by Birkmayer and Mentasti[16], Siegfried and colleagues[39], and Tissot and associates[43]. This point will be more important if ever a margin of safety is required based on animal toxicology studies.

The experience now obtained from 4 centres using Ro 4-4602 and elsewhere[22] with a similar inhibitor (alpha methyldopa hydrazine; MK-485, Merck Sharp & Dohme) permits the conclusion that combining levodopa with an inhibitor of peripheral dopa decarboxylase constitutes a useful advance in the therapy of Parkinson's disease.

The authors would like to express their appreciation for the help and understanding given throughout this study by the Department of Health and Welfare, Ottawa, and the Food and Drug Directorate of Canada.

References

1. Barbeau, A.: *Biochemistry of Parkinson's disease.* Societa Grafica Romana Rome, *2*, 925–927, 1961.
2. Barbeau, A.: L-*Dopa therapy in Parkinson's disease. A critical review of nine years' experience.* Canad. Med. Ass. J., *101*, 791–800, 1969.
3. Barbeau, A.: *Dopamine and blood pressure regulation.* Clin. Res., *17*, 634, 1969.
4. Barbeau, A.: L-*Dopa and juvenile Huntington's disease.* Lancet, *2*, 1066, 1969.
5. Barbeau, A.: *Traitement de la maladie de Parkinson par la L-DOPA.* Un. Med. Canada, *98*, 183–186, 1969.

6. Barbeau, A. – Friesen, H.: *Treatment of Wilson's disease with L-dopa after failure with penicillamine.* Lancet, *1*, 1180–1181, 1970.
7. Barbeau, A. – Gillo-Joffroy, L.: *Treatment of Parkinson's disease with L-dopa and Ro 4-4602, (N DL seryl-N-2 3 4-tri-hydroxybenzylhydrazine).* Excerpta Medica Foundation, Amsterdam, I.C.S. No. 193, p. 171, 1969.
8. Barbeau, A. – Gillo-Joffroy, L. – Boucher, R. – Nowaczynski, W. – Genest, J.: *Renaldosterone system in Parkinson's disease.* Science, *165*, 291–292, 1969.
9. Barbeau, A. – Gillo-Joffroy, L. – Mars, H.: *Therapy of Parkinson's disease with levodopa alone or in association with a peripheral dopa-decarboxylase inhibitor—a comparative study.* New Eng. J. Med., 1970. (Submitted for publication.)
10. Barbeau, A. – Mars, H. – Gillo-Joffroy, L.: *Beneficial and adverse clinical side effects of L-DOPA treatment,* in McDowell, F. H., and Markham, C. H., editors: *Recent advances in Parkinson's disease.* Philadelphia, 1971, F. A. Davis Company. In press.
11. Barbeau, A. – Murphy, G. F. – Sourkes, T. L.: *Excretion of dopamine in diseases of basal ganglia.* Science, *133*, 1706–1707, 1961.
12. Barbeau, A. – Sourkes, T. L. – Murphy, G. F.: *Les catécholamines dans la maladie de Parkinson* in de Ajuriaguerra, J., editor: *Monoamines et systéme nerveux central.* Paris, 1962, Masson et Cie., p. 247.
13. Bartholini, G. – Burkard, W. R. – Pletscher, A. – Bates, H. M.: *Increase of cerebral catecholamines caused by 3,4-dihydroxyphenylalanine after inhibition of peripheral decarboxylase.* Nature, *215*, 852–853, 1967.
14. Bertrand, C. – Martinez, N.: *An apparatus and technique for surgery of dyskinesias.* Neurochirurgia, *2*, 36–46, 1959.
15. Birkmayer, W. – Hornykeiwicz, O.: [*The L-3,4-dihydroxyphenylalanine (DOPA)-effect in Parkinson akinesia*]. Wien. Klin. Wschr., *73*, 877–788, 1961.
16. Birkmayer, W. – Mentasti, M.: *Weitere experimentelle Untersuchungen über den Catecholaminstoffwechsel bei extrapyramidalen Erkrankungen (Parkinson und Chorea-Syndrom).* Arch. Psychiat. Nervenkr., *210*, 29–35, 1967.
17. Calne, D. B. – Spiers, A. S. D. – Stern, G. M. – Laurence, D. T.: *L-Dopa in idiopathic parkinsonism.* Lancet, *2*, 973–976, 1969.
18. Charcot, J. M.: In Bourneville, A., editor: *Lecons sur les désordres du systeme nerveux faites à la Salpétrière Paris, 1892.* Delahaye and Lecrosnier, pp. 155–157.
19. Constantinidis, J. – Bartholini, G. – Tissot, R. – Pletscher, A.: *Accumulation of dopamine in the parenchyma after decarboxylase inhibition in the capillaries of brain,* Experientia, *24*, 130–131, 1968.
20. Constantinidis, J. – de Ajuriaguerra, J.: *Syndrome familial avec tremblement Parkinsonien et anosmie, et sa thérapeutique par la L-DOPA associée à un inhibiteur de la decarboxylase.* Sem. Hop. Paris, *46*, 263–269, 1970.
21. Cooper, I. S.: *Intracerebral injection of procaine into the globus pallidus in hyperkinetic disorders.* Science, *119*, 417–418, 1954.
22. Cotzias, G. C. – Papavasiliou, P. S. – Gellene, R.: *Modification of Parkinsonism-chronic treatment with L-dopa.* New Eng. J. Med., *280*, 337–345, 1969.
23. Cotzias, G. C. – Van Woert, M. H. – Schiffer, L. M.: *Aromatic amino acids and modification of Parkinsonism.* New Eng. J. Med., *276*, 374–379, 1967.
24. Dery, J. P. – De Groot, J. A. – Laurin, C. – Barbeau, A.: [*Anti-Parkinsonian agents. I. New method of objective evaluation of rigidity and tremor in Parkinson's disease*]. Un. Med. Canada, *91*, 842, 847, 1962.
25. Domenjoz, R.: *Parpanit ein neuss Therapeuticum bei Störungen der extrapyramidalen notorik,* Schweiz, Med. Wschr., *76*, 1282–1286, 1946.
26. Ehringer, H. – Hornykiewicz, O.: [*Distribution of noradrenaline and dopamine (3-hydroxytyramine) in the human brain and their behaviour in diseases of the extrapyramidal system*]. Klin. Wschr., *38*, 1236–1239, 1960.

27. Hornykiewicz, O.: *Dopamine (3-hydroxytyramine) and brain function.* Pharmacol. Rev., *18*, 925–964, 1966.
28. Joubert, M. – Barbeau, A.: *Akinesia in Parkinson's disease,* in Barbeau, A., and Brunette, J. R., editors: *Progress in neuro-genetics.* Excerpta Medica Foundation, Amsterdam, 1969, I.C.S. No. 175, pp. 366–376.
29. Joubert, M. – Barbeau, A.: *Methode de mesure de l'akinésie,* Un. Med. Canada, *95*, 531–535, 1955.
30. Kaufmann, W. – Butz, P. – Wiesendanger, M.: *Effekt einer kombinierten Behandlung von Parkinsonpatienten mit l-Dopa und einem Decarboxylasehemmer (Ro 4-4602). Quantitative Analyse der Bradykinesie mittels Reactionszeitmessungen.* Deutsch. Z. Nervenheilk., *197*, 85–100, 1970.
31. Krayenbuhl, H. – Siegfried, J.: *Traitement dé là maladie de Parkinson: L-DOPA ou stéréotaxie.* Neurochirurgie, *16*, 71–76, 1970.
32. Kuchel, O. – Cuche, J. L. – Barbeau, A. – Boucher, R. – Genest, J.: *The urinary ratio of dopamine/norepinephrine (DA:NE) and of noreprinephrine/epinephrine (NE:E) upon assuming upright posture in normal and hypertensive subjects.* Clin. Res. *17*, 645, 1969.
33. Mars, H. – Libman, L. – Schwartz, A. – Gillo-Joffrey, L. – Barbeau, A.: *L-DOPA in Parkinson's disease. Results of a co-operative study in the Montreal area.* Canad. J. Psychiat., 1971. In press.
34. McDowell, F. – Lee, J. E. – Swift, T. – Sweet, R. D. – Ogsbury, J. S. – Kessler, J. T.: *Treatment of Parkinson's syndrome with L-dihydroxyphenylalanine (levodopa).* Ann. Intern. Med., *72*, 29–35, 1970.
35. Pletscher, A. – Gey, K. F. – Burkard, W. P.: *Besinflussung des cerebralen Stoffwechsels von 5-Hydroxytryptamin durch Decarboxylasehemmung.* Helv. Physiol. Pharmacol. Acta, *21*, C46–C50, 1963.
36. Schwab, R. S. – England, A. C. – Poskanzer, D. C. – Young, R. R.: *Amantadine in the treatment of Parkinson's disease.* J. A. M. A., *208*, 1168–1170, 1969.
37. Siegfired, J.: *Traitement du Parkinsonisme avec la L-DOPA associée à un inhibiteur de la décarboxylase.* Med. Hyg., *27*, 543–545, 1969.
38. Siegfried, J. – Klaiber, R. – Perret, E. – Ziegler, W. H.: *The treatment of Parkinsons's disease with L-dopa combined with a decarboxylase inhibitor.* Excerpta Medica Foundation, Amsterdam, 1969, I.C.S. No. 193, p. 171.

   Perret, E.: *Treatment of Parkinsonism with L-DOPA in association with decarboxylase inhibitor.* Pharmacologia Clin., *2*, 23–26, 1969.
40. Sigwald, J. – Bovet, D. – Dumont, G.: *Le traitement de la maladie de Parkinson par le chlorhydrate de diethylaminoethyl-N-thiodiphenylamine (2987 R.P.).* Premiers resultats, Rev. Neurol., *78*, 581–584, 1946.
41. Spiegel, E. A. – Wycis, H. T. – Marks, M. – Lee, A. J.: *Stereotaxic apparatus for operations on the human brain.* Science, *106*, 349–350, 1947.
42. Tissot, R. – Bartholini, G. – Pletscher, A.: *Drug-induced changes of extracerebral dopa metabolism in man.* Arch. Neurol., *20*, 187–190, 1969.
43. Tissot, R. – Gaillard, J. M. – Guggisberg, M. – Gauthier, G. – de Ajuriaguerra, J.: *Thérapeutique du syndrome de Parkinson par la L-Dopa "per os" associée à un inhibiteur de la décarboxylase (Ro IV 46.02).* Presse Med., *77*, 619–622, 1969.
44. Voller, G. W. – Deze, J. – Gundlach, U.: *Treatment of Parkinson's disease with levodopa.* Med. Welt., *21*, 409–411, 1970.
45. Yahr, M. D. – Duvoisin, R. C. – Schear, M. J. – Barrett, R. E. – Hoehn, M.M.: *Treatment of Parkinsonism with levodopa.* Arch. Neurol., *21*, 343–354, 1969.

Part 11

Metabolic and Biochemical Actions

This selection of key papers on the development, use and understanding of levodopa in Parkinsonism collects together those reports describing the most important original observations.

When we consider the metabolic and biochemical aspects however, it is impossible to single out individual papers which can be regarded as of paramount importance in their own right, or any key group of scientists whose work has provided a basis for the total research effort. Our present knowledge depends on the sum of a large number of observations from groups working in different parts of the world. Among these should be mentioned the teams surrounding Blaschko, Udenfriend, Sourkes, Hornykiewicz and Sandler.

*With so many separate observations it is invidious to single out any one paper and a recent general review has been selected (Calne D. B., and Sandler M., Nature, **226**, 21, 1970), partly because of the clarity of its expression and partly because the two authors have made important contributions to both the clinical and biochemical studies.*

Their metabolic diagram is particularly relevant even though the paper in now includes a critically selected bibliography, but its greatest merit lies in the summary of the knowledge of the biochemistry and metabolism of levodopa. Their metabolic diagram is particularly relevant even though the paper is now almost three years old. The paper draws particular attention to the many compounds that can be formed after levodopa administration. It thus stresses that the therapeutic action of levodopa may not stem from dopamine repletion of striatal nerve endings.

However, though the most obvious biochemical effect of levodopa administra-

143

tion is the increase in brain dopamine and the other metabolites, it must be emphasised that other biochemical effects occur and could mediate the therapeutic effect. Among these may be mentioned: increase in cerebrospinal fluid 5-hydroxyindoleacetic acid and reduction in brain serotonin; decreased 5-adenosylmethionine (which is essential to the ortho methylation pathway for catecholomine inactivation); modification of brain cholinergic mechanisms. Many of these were brought out at a recent symposium (Neurology, 22, Supp. 72–102, 1972).

Moreover Sandler and his co-workers (Sandler M., Carter S. B., Hunter K. R., and Stern G. M., Nature, 241, 439, 1973) have shown that patients receiving levodopa may form pharmacologically active tetrahydrosoquinoline alkaloids.

Reprinted from D. B. Calne and M. Sandler, Nature, **226**, *21, 1970, by kind permission of the authors and MacMillan Journals Ltd.*

L-DOPA AND PARKINSONISM

D. B. CALNE AND M. SANDLER
ROYAL POSTGRADUATE MEDICAL SCHOOL AND
QUEEN CHARLOTTE'S MATERNITY HOSPITAL

During the past decade a new approach to Parkinsonism has evolved, culminating in the introduction of L-dopa (short for L-dihydroxy-phenylalanine), a drug which is likely to have an important impact on future management of this syndrome. Treatment had previously been unrewarding. There had been no important development in drug therapy for a century and the long-term benefits of stereo-tactic surgery have failed to confirm all the initial enthusiastic claims.

Parkinsonism is a chronic neurological disorder characterised by tremor, rigidity of the limbs and poverty of movement (hypokinesia). In most patients, initial symptoms develop in the fifth or sixth decade of life and gradually progress, death usually occuring about ten years after onset. Parkinsonism is common, its estimated prevalence being 1 in 1,000 of the population.

Known causes of Parkinsonism include viral infection (encephalitis lethargia), toxins (manganese , carbon monoxide), vascular disease (atherosclerosis) and drugs (phenothiazines, haloperidol, reserpine). In most cases, however, no cause can be identified. Pathological examination of the brain reveals widespread degenerative changes in the basal ganglia, particularly the substantia nigra and corpus striatum.

Pharmacological considerations

The introduction of reserpine as an antihypertensive agent in 1954 was soon followed by the recognition of Parkinsonism as a dose-dependent side effect. Reserpine depletes the tissues of catecholamines and 5-hydroxytrypamine. Dopamine, the most important catecholamine in this context, is widespread in the body, its concentration in various tissues depending on species. In the brain, high concentrations are localised in the striatum, where concentrations of noradrenaline are low. Hornykiewicz and his colleagues [1,2] examined brains obtained at autopsy from patients with idiopathic and postencephalitic Parkinsonism and noted gross depletion of striatal dopamine; the concentration of homovanillic acid, the major metabolite of dopamine, is similarly reduced in the brain[2] and cerebrospinal fluid[3,4,5] of Parkinsonian patients.

Dopamine was initially thought to act merely as a precursor in the synthesis of noradrenaline and adrenaline, but in 1957 Blaschko[6] suggested that it might have some regulating functions of its own. Two years later, Carlsson[7] proposed that it might be a neurotransmitter in the central nervous system. Accumulating evidence supports this view. Histochemical fluorescence techniques have revealed the presence of dopamine in cell bodies of the substantia nigra and in nerve endings of the corpus striatum[8]. Dense granular vesicles probably containing dopamine are present in the terminal boutons of striatal nerve endings[9]. Experimental lesions of the brain stem cause depletion of striatal dopamine[10]. Stimulation of the substantia nigra leads to an increase in dopamine collected from a cannula in the putamen[11] and provokes a corresponding increase in the concentration of homovanillic acid in the cerebrospinal fluid[12,13]. The action of dopamine applied to neurones in the caudate nucleus has been investigated by microelectrophoresis with multibarrelled pipettes[14,15] and inhibition has been recorded in some 60 per cent of cells. Inhibition of caudate neurones has also been demonstrated following stimulation of the substantia nigra[16,17]. All these findings support the conclusion that dopamine is a synaptic transmitter, and suggest that it is concerned with mediating inhibition in a nigrostriatral pathway. The present view is that the therapeutic activity of L-dopa in Parkinsonism derives from its conversion to dopamine in the brain.

Other findings indicate that acetylcholine may be an excitatory transmitter in the striatum[18,19]. Drugs which block the muscarinic effects of acetylcholine in the central nervous system have formed the basis of anti-Parkinsonian therapy since they were introduced by

Charcot a century ago. It seems that a balance may exist between the activity of acetylcholine and dopamine in the striatum. In Parkinsonism, there seems to be disequilibrium in the direction of cholinergic dominance[20,21]. Drugs which deplete the brain of dopamine (for example, reserpine) or increase the concentration of acetylcholine (for example, physostigmine) exacerbate Parkinsonism[22]. Conversely, drugs which reduce cholinergic function (atropine) or enhance dopaminergic activity (L-dopa) are beneficial.

An alternative mechanism of action for anticholinergic agents has been suggested recently[23]. Studies on isolated synaptosomes suggest that these drugs may inhibit re-uptake of dopamine at nerve endings, so that higher concentrations persist in the region of the synapse.

Biochemical considerations

Although the principal biosynthetic pathway of catecholamine metabolism was proposed by Blaschko in 1939[24], the first and rate-limiting step[23] in the route from L-tyrosine to dopamine was characterised quite recently[26] (the D forms of amino-acids seem to occur only rarely in nature). The responsible enzyme, tryosine hydroxylase, possesses a K_m such that it is normally likely to be saturated in relation to its substrate, tyrosine[27]. Thus the reaction cannot be "driven" and it probably follows that Parkinsonism cannot be effectively treated by feeding an excess of L-tyrosine.

L-Dopa is avidly decarboxylated in most species by the relatively non-specific L-dopa decarboxylase[28] which is now known to consist of several isoenzymes[29]. Decarboxylase activity has been surprisingly difficult to demonstrate in the human brain[30]. If decarboxylation proves to be the rate-limiting step in the formation of dopamine at this site rather than tryosine hydroxylation[30], important questions will be raised in relation to the therapeutic action of L-dopa in Parkinsonism. It is even possible that transamination, which is known to be a minor pathway in the metabolic disposal of L-dopa[31], assumes a more important role within the brain. Direct O-methylation of L-dopa is another of many possible routes yet to be studied which may be important during therapy[32]. But in view of the consistent finding of high L-dopa decarboxylase activity in the central nervous system of other mammalian species, it seems possible that the problems encountered in demonstrating the human enzyme are technical.

L-dopa gains ready access to the central nervous system[33], unlike the catecholamines which do not cross the blood-brain barrier with any facility[34]. There is no such barrier to certain compounds bearing a structural resemblance to dopamine, such as apomorphine; this drug possesses some pharmacological properties similar to dopamine and might have played a useful part in the treatment of Parkinsonism[35,36], were it not for the severe nausea and vomiting which it provokes. It is possible that related "dopamine substitutes" may soon be evolved.

Because L-dopa decarboxylase is so widespread outside the central nervous system, considerably larger doses of L-dopa than might otherwise have been necessary must be given to surmount peripheral decarboxylating mechanisms and, after passing through the blood-brain barrier, generate a therapeutic concentration of dopamine within the brain. Peripheral production of dopamine may be responsible for the cardiovascular side effects observed in some patients. An attempt has been made to control these reactions and reduce the dose of L-dopa by adding decarboxylase inhibitors[37] which do not penetrate the blood-brain barrier[38]; it is too early to assess the value of these drugs.·

A proportion of the dopamine produced in the body is converted to noradrenaline by dopamine β-hydroxylase[39]. Although inhibition of the enzyme might seem a rational approach to treatment of Parkinsonism, it is likely that only a very small proportion of orally administered L-dopa eventually undergoes β-hydroxylation, for there is only a marginal increase of noradrenaline metabolites in the urine after treatment[31]. The position is complicated by the possibility of a decreased conversion of dopamine to noradrenaline in Parkinsonian subjects[40]. L-dopa may induce a localised but highly significant increase in noradrenaline in certain regions of the brain, with only minimal changes in the pattern of its urinary metabolites. The amino-acid, *threo*-dihydroxyphenylserine (DOPS), not usually present in the body, is decarboxylated to noradrenaline[41] without intermediate formation of dopamine. Administration of DOPS to reserpinised animals[42] and a limited study in Parkinsonian patients[41] have failed to achieve any therapeutic response. It is therefore unlikely that changes in noradrenaline concentration are relevant to the improvement induced by L-dopa.

Apart from its conversion to noradrenaline, dopamine may be degraded by O-methylation or oxidative deamination (Fig. 1).

These and related pathways have been the subject of a recent detailed review[44]. Oxidative deamination is likely to be of major importance in the brain, and dopamine is known to be an excellent substrate for the responsible enzyme, monoamine oxidase (MAO)[15]. Human brain MAO consists of four isoenzymes, each with its own characteristic substrate and inhibitor specificity[46], and one such isoenzyme, termed MAO_4, has a particular affinity for dopamine; of all brain areas investigated, the highest specific activity of this isoenzyme for dopamine as substrate was found in the basal ganglia. Although previous attempts to alleviate Parkinsonism with MAO inhibitors have resulted in only limited improvement[3], an inhibitor tailored to this particular isoenzyme might stand more chance of therapeutic success.

The intermediate aldehyde formed by oxidative deamination of dopamine is largely oxidised to the corresponding acid, although a small amount is reduced to the alcohol (Fig. 1.) The acid, dihydroxyphenylacetic acid, may be 3-O-methylated to homovanillic acid. Large amounts of both acids, quantitatively the most important metabolic end products, are excreted in the urine after administration of L-dopa to Parkinsonian patients[31].

By using quantitative gas chromatographic procedures[48,49], it has been possible to obtain information about various minor metabolic routes[31]. These observations may be important, for there is a discrepancy between the time course of the therapeutic response to orally administered L-dopa, which is usually slow, and the generation of dopamine within the central nervous system, which is rapid. Although it has been tacitly assumed that clinical improvement stems from the formation of dopamine in the brain, there are other possibilities. Part of the clinical effect may derive from a slow accumulation within the central nervous system of some minor metabolite unconnected with the principal route of degradation of L-dopa.

One group of compounds which may be important is the *m*-hydroxylated amines. The comparatively large increase in the quantity of urinary *m*-hydroxyphenylacetic acid excreted after oral administration of L-dopa[31] is a result of *p*-dehydroxylation by gut flora, for it can be decreased by a small concomitant dose of neomycin[50]. In view of the known pharmacological action of *m*-tyrosine[51], this type of compound could play some part in the therapeutic action of L-dopa.

149

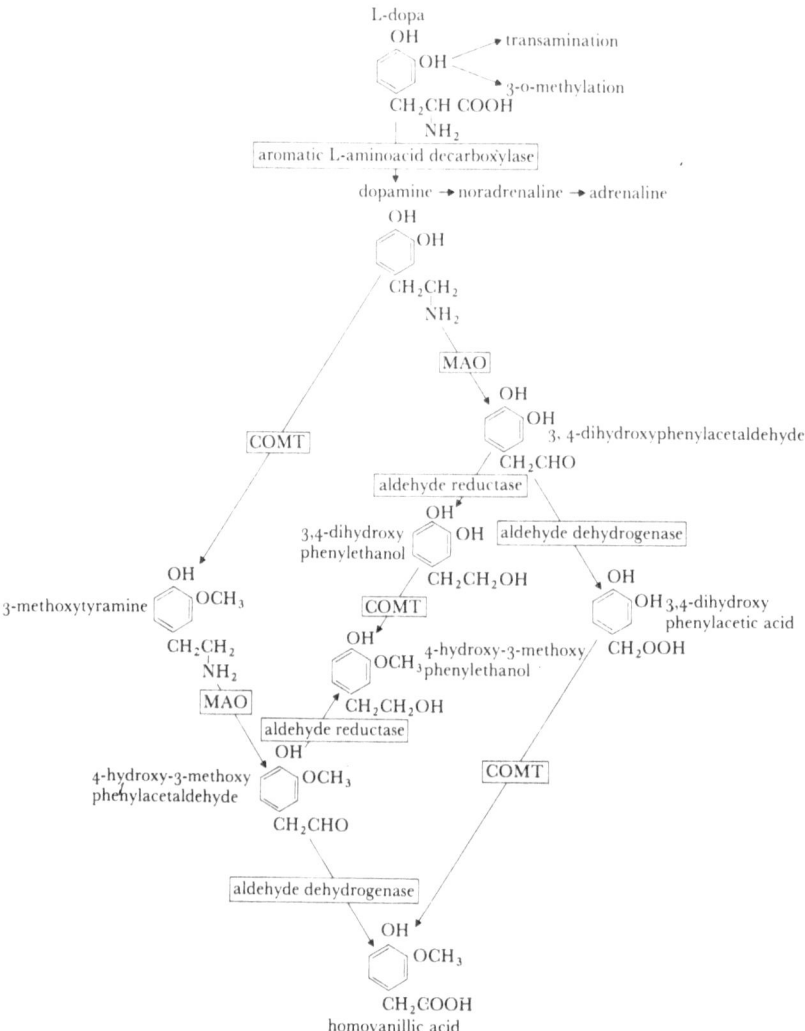

Figure 1. Metabolic pathways of L-dopa. MAO, Monoamine oxidase; COMT, catechol O-methyltransferase

Single-ring compounds with a 2,4,5-substitution pattern seem to have high psychotomimetic activity[52]. Attention has recently been drawn[53] to two ways in which this type of compound might be produced in Parkinsonian patients: first by a possible action of p-hydroxyphenylpyruvate oxidase on dihydroxyphenylpyruvic acid generated in increased amounts by transamination[31], and second —of considerably greater potential importance—by 6-hydroxylation of dopamine itself to form 6-hydroxydopamine (2,4,5-trihydroxy-phenylethylamine)[54]. Administration of this compound to animals can produce a "chemical sympathectomy"[55] or bring about degeneration of central neurones[56]. Patients on long-term therapy with L-dopa display certain features of blockade of the sympathetic nervous system[57], and although this is probably a transient pharmacological effect, the possibility of some permanent damage by 6-hydroxydopamine has not been excluded. Orthostatic hypotension may occur in Parkinsonian patients who have never received L-dopa[58], and Sandler[53] has suggested that 6-hydroxydopamine, or a compound similar to it, may be generated endogenously in patients with idiopathic Parkinsonism, causing neuronal degeneration in areas of high dopamine concentration, such as the caudate nucleus. This could provide a biochemical basis for the clinical features of the disease.

Dopamine is not the only amine disturbed in Parkinsonism. There is sometimes a decrease of 5-hydroxytryptamine (5-HT) in the brains of affected subjects. Treatment with the 5-HT precursor, 5-hydroxytryptophan (5-HTP), suppresses some of the physical signs in certain Parkinson-like states in experimental animals[59]. Although this cannot be achieved in human Parkinsonism, there have been occasional accounts[60] of 5-HTP producing dramatic improvement when L-dopa has failed.

Clinical studies

In 1961, Hornykiewicz reported favourable results following intravenous administration of 50–150 mg. of L-dopa to twenty Parkinsonian patients[61]; similar observations were made independently after oral administration to six patients (paper presented at International Congress of Neurology, 1961, by A. Barbeau). Therapeutic effects are not easy to evaluate in Parkinsonism because of rapid spontaneous fluctuations. Thus conflicting accounts began to appear.

Although initial observations were supported by several subsequent studies, less favourable findings were also recorded, as reviewed by Barbeau[62].

All these investigations involved administration of small doses of L-dopa for short periods. In 1967, Cotzias and his colleagues[63] achieved large oral dose regimens for periods of up to a year by gradually increasing the intake of dopa, titrating this against adverse effects in each patient individually. DL-Dopa was used at that time because it is cheaper than the separated L-isomer and doses up to 16 g/day were reached (equivalent to 8 g/day of L-dopa). Dramatic therapeutic results were obtained in eight out of sixteen patients. Four developed transient granulocytopenia. Subsequent studies with the pure L-isomer have shown that the same impressive therapeutic response can be obtained with far less risk of bone marrow depression[62,64,47]. There is remarkable consistency in the results obtained at different centres. All reports using the technique of slowly increasing dosage introduced by Cotzias *et al.*[63] confirm the general conclusion that in a considerable proportion of patients L-dopa is a far more potent therapeutic agent than any previously available. It is not known why some patients fail to benefit even from a relatively large dose. It may be that absorption from the alimentary tract, normally rapid[74], differs in these subjects, and the effect of dietary factors merits further investigation. For example, pyridoxine, paradoxically a co-factor for L-dopa decarboxylase[28], antagonises the beneficial effect of L-dopa (paper presented at International Congress of Neurology, 1969, by R. C. Duvoisin, M. D. Yahr, M. J. Schear, M. M. Hoehn and R. E. Barrett), perhaps because of Schiff's base formation.

Idiopathic and postencephalitic Parkinsonism both respond to L-dopa. Parkinsonism due to manganese toxicity is also improved[60], an observation in accord with recent reports that striatal dopamine is depleted in this condition in both man (paper presented at International Congress of Neurology, 1969, by H. Bernheimer, W. Birkmayer, O. Hornykiewicz, K. Jellinger and F. Seitelberger) and experimental animals[75]. Patients with severe, long standing Parkinsonism seem to tolerate L-dopa less well than mildly affected cases of recent origin, although therapeutic successes and failures occur at every grade of severity. It is likely, however, that at least 50 per cent of the total Parkinsonian population may obtain benefit from L-dopa and in some patients the improvement will be substantial. The principal clinical feature to improve is hypokinesia, which is probably the most important single functional disturbance in Parkinsonism. The more obvious and less disabling tremor and rigidity are also alleviated but less consistently. When treatment with L-dopa stops, patients return to their pretreatment status. At present there is insufficient evidence to draw any conclusions as to whether the gradual downhill course of Parkinsonian patients is modified by L-dopa.

Although normal subjects receiving substantial doses of L-dopa apparently experience few symptoms apart from gastrointestinal effects[76], numerous dose-dependent adverse reactions to similar drug dosage have been reported in Parkinsonian subjects. Several, such as nausea and orthostatic hypotension, can usually be overcome by slowing the rate of increase in dose. Other side effects, such as dyskinesia and delusions, are less easy to manage and may prove so troublesome that treatment has to be abandoned. One aspect of L-dopa therapy which has recently been publicised is a claim that an increase in libido may be induced. Any drug which ameliorates a chronic disease is likely to enhance all forms of activity and a specific aphrodisiac action has not been demonstrated. All adverse reactions to L-dopa so far encountered have disappeared when treatment has stopped, and there have been no deaths directly attributable to this drug.

Further problems

Chronic degenerative diseases of the central nervous system are likely to result in complex changes in the mechanisms of synthesis and inactivation of transmitters. In addition, such phenomena as denervation sensitivity may take place at the receptors. Flooding the brain with high concentrations of the precursor of a transmitter is likely to result in even more complex functional alterations. For example, L-dopa probably competes with tryptophan for tissue transport mechanisms and with 5-HTP for decarboxylation; the depletion of brain 5-HT observed after administration of L-dopa[77] probably derives from a variety of such causes.

The analysis of these and similar effects of L-dopa poses a considerable task for neuropharmacologists, but it seems possible that important therapeutic advances will depend on their clarification. Other approaches which may prove useful include investigation of interactions between L-dopa and other drugs which may potentiate its actions in the central nervous system. Anticholinergic agents[23], amphetamine[35] and amantadine[78] are of interest in this context.

Perhaps the most important point arising from these studies is the realisation that striking therapeutic results can be obtained by a new approach to chronic diseases of the nervous system. Previous investigations have focused attention on physiological and pathological abnormalities, but it now seems that neuropharmacological disturbances ought to receive more emphasis. Attempts to modulate the action of transmitters in the central nervous system have already achieved some success in psychiatric illness. The therapeutic results currently being attained in Parkinsonism suggest that similar approaches might be justifiable for other chronic degenerative diseases of the central nervous system.

References

1. Ehringer, H. – Hornykiewicz, O. Klin. Wschr., *38*, 1236, 1960.
2. Hornykiewicz, O.: Pharmacol. Revs., *18*, 925, 1966.
3. Bernheimer, H. – Birkmayer, W. – Hornykiewicz, O.: Wien. Klin. Wschr., *78*, 417, 1966.
4. Galdberg, H. – Turner, J. – Hanieh, A. – Ashcroft, G. – Crawford, T. B. B. – Gillingham, F. J.: Confin. Neurol., *29*, 73, 1967.
5. Johansson, B. – Roos, B. E.: Life Sci., *6*, 1449, 1967.
6. Blaschko, H.: Experientia, *13*, 9, 1957.
7. Carlsson, A.: Pharmacol. Rev., *11*, 490, 1959.
8. Hillarp, N.-A. – Fuxe, K. – Dahlstrom, A.: In *Mechanisms of Release of Biogenic Amines*. Edit. by von Euler, U. S., Rossell, S., and Uvnas, B., *5*, 31. Wenner-Gren Centre International Symposium Series (Pergamon, Oxford, 1966).
9. Hokfelt, T.: Z. Zellforsch., *91*, 1, 1968.
10. Poirier, L. J. – Sourkes, T. L.: Brain, *88*, 181, 1965.
11. McLennan, H.: Experientia, *21*, 725, 1965.
12. Portig, P. J. – Vogt, M.: J. Physiol, *204*, 687, 1969.
13. Bloom, F. E. – Costa, E. – Salmoiraghi, G. C.: J. Pharmacol. Exp. Ther., *150*, 244, 1965.
14. McLennan, H. – York, D. H.: J. Physiol., *189*, 393, 1967.
15. Connor, J. D.: Science, *160*, 899, 1968.
16. Feltz, P.: J. Physiol., *205*, SP, 1969.
17. McLennan, H. – York, D. H.: J. Physiol., *187*, 163, 1966.
18. Gallindo, A. – Krnjevic, K. – Schwartz, S.: J. Physiol., *192*, 359, 1967.
19. McGeer, P. L. – Boulding, J. E. – Gibson, W. C. – Foulkes, R. G.: J. Amer. Med. Assoc., *177*, 665, 1961.
20. Barbeau, A.: Canad. Med. Ass. J., *87*, 802, 1962.
21. Arvidsson, J. – Roos, B.-E. – Steg, G.: Acta Physiol. Scand., *67*, 398, 1966.
22. Duvoisin, R.: Arch. Neurol., *17*, 124, 1967.
23. Coyle, J. T. – Snyder, S. H.: Science, *166*, 899, 1960.

24. Blaschko, H.: J. Physiol., *96*, 50P, 1939.
25. Udenfriend, S.: Pharmacol. Rer., *18*, 43, 1966.
26. Nagatsu, T. – Levitt, M. – Udenfriend, S.: J. Biol. Chem., *239*, 2010, 1964.
27. Peters, D. A. V. – McGeer, P. L. – McGeer, E. G.: J. Neurochem., *15*, 1431, 1968.
28. Sourkes, T. L.: Pharmacol. Rev., *18*, 53, 1966.
29. Coulson, W. F. – Bender, D. A. – Jepson, J. B.; Biochem. J., *115*, 63P, 1969.
30. Robins, E. – Robins, J. M. – Croninger, A. B. – Moses, S. G. – Spencer, S. J. – Hughes, R. W.: Biochem. Med., *1*, 240. 1967.
31. Calne, D. B. – Karoum, F. – Ruthven, C. R. J. – Sandler, M.: Brit. J. Pharmacol., *37*, 57, 1969.
32. Tissot, R. – Bartholini, G. – Pletscher, A.; Arch. Neurol., *20*, 187, 1969.
33. Holtz, P.: Pharmacol. Rev., *11*, 317, 1959.
34. Weil-Malherbe, H.: In *Adrenergic Mechanisms*. Edit. by Vane, J. R., Wolstenholme, G. E. W., and O'Connor, M., 421. (Churchill, London, 1960).
35. Ernst, A. M.: Acta Physiol. Pharmacol. Neurl., *15*, 141, 1969.
36. Cotzias, G. C. – Papavasiliou, P. S. – Fehling, C. – Kaufman, B. – Mena, I.: New Engl. J. Med., *282*, 31, 1970.
37. Tissot, R. – Gaillard, J. M. – Guggisberg, M. – Gauthier, G. – de Ajuriaguerra, J.: Presse Med., *77*, 619, 1969.
38. Bartholini, G. – Pletscher, A.: J. Pharmacol. Exp. Ther., *161*, 14, 1968.
39. Levin, E. Y. – Levenberg, B. – Kaufman, S.: J. Biol. Chem., *235*, 2080, 1960.
40. Goodall, McC. – Alton, H.: J. Clin. Invest., *48*, 2300, 1969.
41. Kirshner, N.: Pharmacol. Rev., *11*, 350, 1959.
42. Hornykiewicz, O. – Davidson, L. – Kraster, F.: *Proc. Fourth Intern. Cong. Pharmacol.*, Basle, *71*, 1969.
43. Hornykiewicz, O.: *Proc. Second Intern. Pharmacol.* Meeting, Prague. Edit. by Raskova, H., *2*, 57 (Pergamon, Oxford, 1964).
44. Sandler, M. – Ruthven, C. R. J.: In *Progress of Medicinal Chemistry*. Edit. by Ellis, G. P., and West, G. B., *6*, 200 (Butterworth, London, 1969).
45. Weiner, N.: Arch. Biochem. Biophys., *91*, 182, 1960.
46. Collins, G. G. S. – Sandler, M. – Williams, E. D. – Youdim, M. B. H.: Nature, *225*, 817, 1970.
47. Barbeau, A. – Duchastel, Y.: Canad. Psychiat. Assoc. J., *7*, 591, 1962.
48. Karoum, F. – Ruthven, C. R. J., Sandler, M. – Clin. Chim. Acta, *20*, 427, 1968.
49. Karoum, F. – Anah, C. O. – Ruthven, C. R. J. – Sandler, M.: Clin. Chim. Acta, *24*, 341, 1969.
50. Sandler, M. – Karoum, F. – Ruthven, C. R. J. – Calne, D. B.: Science, *166*, 1417, 1969.
51. Blaschko, H. – Chrusciel, T. L.: J. Physiol., *151*, 272, 1960.
52. Shulgin, A. T. – Sargent, T. – Naranjo, C.: Nature, *221*, 537, 1969.
53. Sandler, M.: *Proc. Laurentian Meeting on Dopa in Parkinsonism*. (In the press.)
54. Senoh, S. – Creveling, C. R. – Udenfriend, S. – Witkop, B.: J. Amer. Chem. Soc., *81*, 6236, 1959.
55. Thoenen, H. – Tranzer, J. P.: Naunyn-Schmiedebergs Arch. Pharmak., *261*, 271, 1968.
56. Ungerstedt, U.: Europ. J. Phtrmacol., *5*, 107, 1968.
57. Calne, D. B. – Brennan, J. – Spiers, A. S. D. – Stern, G. M.: Brit. Med. J., *1*, 474, 1970.
58. Shy, G. M. – Drager, G. A.: Arch. Neurol., *2*, 511, 1960.
59. Goldstein, M. – Battista, A. F. – Nakatani, S. – Anagnoste, B.: Nature, *224*, 382, 1969.

60. Mena, I. – Court, J. – Fuenzalida, S – Papavasiliou, P. S. – Cotzias, G. C.:
    New Engl. J. Med., *282*, 5, 1970.
61. Birkmayer, W. – Hornykiewicz, O.: Wien. Klin. Wschr., *73*, 787, 1961. *224*,
62. Barbeau, A.: Canad. Med. Assoc. J., *101*, 791, 1969.
63. Cotzias, G. C. – van Woert, M. H. – Schiffer, L. M.: New Engl. J. Med.,
    276, 374, 1967.
64. Cotzias, G. C. – Papavasiliou, P. S. – Gellene, R. – Aronson, R. B.: Trans.
    Assoc. Amer. Physicians, *81*, 171, 1968.
65. Cotzias, G. C. – Papavasiliou, P. S. – Gellene, R.: New Engl. J. Med., *280*,
    337, 1969.
66. Yahr, M. D. – Duvoisin, R. C. – Hoehn, M. M. – Schear, M. J. – Barrett,
    R. E.: Trans. Amer. Neurol. Assoc., *93*, 56, 1968.
67. Yahr, M. D. – Duvoisin, R. C. – Schear, M. J. – Barrett, R. E. – Hoehn,
    M. M.: Arch. Neurol., *21*, 343, 1969.
68. Calne, D. B. – Stern, G. M. – Laurence, D. R. – Sharkey, J. – Armitage, P.:
    Lancet, i, *744*, 1969.
69. Calne, D. B. – Spiers, A. S. D. – Stern, G. M. – Laurance, D. K. – Armitage, P.
    – Lancet, ii, 1973, 1969.
70. Duvoisin, R. C.: In *Psychotropic Drugs and Dysfunctions of the Basal Ganglia*.
    Edit. by Crane, G. E., and Gardner, R., *135*, (US Govt. Printing Office,
    Washington, 1969).
71. Godwin-Austen, R. B. – Tomlinson, E. B. – Frears, C. C. – Kok, H. W. L.:
    Lancet, ii, *165*, 1969.
72. McDowell, F. – Lee, J. F. – Swift, T. – Sweet, R. D. – Ogsbury, J. S. –
    Kessler, J. J.: Ann. Intern. Med., *72*, 29, 1970.
73. Mawdsley, C.: Brit. Med. J., *1*, 331, 1970.
74. Peaston, M. J. T. – Bianchine, J. R.: Brit, Med. J., *1*, 400, 1970.
75. Neff, N. H. – Barrett, R. E. – Costa, E.: Experientia, *25*, 1140, 1969.
76. Ausel, R. D.: *Proc. Laurentian Meeting on Dopa in Parkinsonism*. (In the press).
77. Bartholini, G. – Pletscher, A. – Burkhard, W. P.: J. Pharm. Pharmacol.,
    20, 228, 1968.
78. Schwab, R. S. – England, A. C. – Poskanzer, D. C. – Young, R. R.: J. Amer.
    Med. Assoc., *208*, 116S, 1969.

Part 12

Further problems

Though big advances have been made during the last few years in both our understanding of the pathophysiology of Parkinsonism and of its therapy with levodopa, it must not be assumed that all the problems are now solved. This applies not only to our understanding of how the existing therapeutic agents work, but also to the establishment of an optimally effective regime.

Several of these problems have already been alluded to in some of the earlier sections but may be summarised here:

The determination of the most appropriate balance and dosage of the various anti-Parkinsonism agents, e.g. levodopa, anti-cholinergics, amantadine.

The long-term assessment of therapy with levodopa with particular reference to the reduced therapeutic effect and the increased incidence of neurological and endocrine side-effects.

More extensive assessment of the merits of decarboxylase inhibitors as a means of increasing the therapeutic effect while reducing side-effects.

A more accurate appraisal of the exact biochemical mode of action of the various agents.

Studies are still continuing and it can be confidently anticipated that further advances in the therapy of Parkinson's syndrome and probably of other degenerative disorders of the nervous system will emerge during the next decade. The life span of levodopa in the therapy of Parkinsonism may in consequence be rather limited and be followed by other drug combinations or different and better compounds. Nevertheless, it must be slressed thal levodopa is at present the most effective single therapeutic agent available.

From the scientific point of view it is to be hoped that when new therapeutic methods are found, they will arise as did levodopa as a rational development from basic research rather than by chance.

Appendix

Current views on the clinical use of levodopa

This review of the use of levodopa in Parkinsonism demonstrates the development of our ideas. The technique in levodopa therapy has changed with increasing experience and a guide to current clinical practice is therefore appended.

Indications for levodopa

Levodopa is effective in most types of Parkinsonism, idiopathic, arteriosclerotic and postencephalitic. It is only very rarely effective in drug induced Parkinsonism. Previous neurosurgery is not a contra-indication to the use of levodopa.

Dosage and method of administration

The dosage and method of administration are variable and must be tailored to the individual patient for the best results. Thus no more than a general guide is possible.

Suggested schedule for hospitalised patients:

Initially 0.25–1.0 g daily in up to five divided doses immediately after food. Dosage should be increased by 0.5–1.0 g every three to four days until adequate improvement results or intolerable side-effects appear. Of severe side-effects appear, the dosage should be gradually decreased to the maximum tolerated. The majority of patients will tolerate the rapid dose increase outlined above, but occasionally intolerance may prevent patients from reaching effective dosage levels. When patients discontinue therapy due to intolerance they should be re-started on 0.25–0.5 g daily in small divided doses, increasing by 0.125–0.5 g at weekly intervals.

Suggested schedule for outpatients and in general practice:

Initially 0.125 g twice daily immediately after food. After one week, the dose may be increased to 0.125 g four or five times daily. Thereafter dosage should be increased at weekly intervals by 0.375 g daily, the total daily dose being given in four or five divided doses. The response of individual patients varies and some patients may tolerate a more rapid rate of increase, e.g. by 0.25–0.5 g daily at intervals of three to four days.

Maintenance therapy

Improvement is usually seen in two to three weeks. The range of dosage at which improvement occurs varies between 2.5 and 8.0 g daily but the majority find 3.0–5.0 g effective. Further improvement is the rule and may occur up to six months or even longer.

When the optimum daily dosage for any particular patient has been reached, it may need to be redistributed throughout the day to meet fluctuations in the individual's requirements. Most patients find a four to five times daily dosage scheme satisfactory; some obtain smoother effect with two-hourly administration; others, who develop akinetic crises at particular times of the day, learn by experience the daily dosage scheme most suited to their needs.

After a period at the maximum tolerated dosage level, side-effects may slowly develop, usually in the form of involuntary movements. These generally regress without loss of therapeutic effect if the dosage is slightly reduced.

Side-effects

Tolerance to levodopa varies widely between patients and is related to the rate of dosage increase. Postencephalitic Parkinsonian patients tolerate the drug less well. Side-effects, usually dose-related, occur at some time in most patients. During the initiation of therapy nausea and vomiting, anorexia, weakness and hypotension, usually postural (but a labile hypertension may rarely be seen) are most frequent. Nausea and vomiting may be minimised by administering levodopa immediately after food; an anti-emetic, e.g. cyclizine hydrochloride 50 mg three times daily may also be helpful. Psychiatric disturbances, including mild elation, depression, anxiety, agitation, aggression, hallucinations and delusions are also encountered. Involuntary movements, commonly in the form of oral dyskinesias, often accompanied by "paddling" foot movements, or of the choreo-athetoid type are most commonly observed with long-term therapy.

Transient rises in SGOT, SGPT and alkaline phosphatase values have been noted; serum uric acid and blood urea nitrogen levels are occasionally increased. On some occasions the urine passed during levodopa treatment may be altered in colour. Usually red-tinged, this will turn dark on standing. These changes are due to metabolites and are no cause for concern.

General precautions and contra-indications

Patients who improve on levodopa therapy should be advised to resume normal activities gradually as rapid mobilisation may increase the risk of injury.

Care should be taken when using levodopa in the following circumstances; in endocrine, renal, hepatic, pulmonary or cardio-vascular disease; particularly where there is a history of myocardial infarction in patients with peptic ulcer; where sympathominetic drugs may be required, e.g. bronchial asthma; where antihypertensive drugs are being used. Periodic evaluation of hepatic, haematopoietic renal and cardiovascular functions are advised.

Levodopa is contra-indicated in narrow-angle glaucoma (it may be used in wide-angle glaucoma provided that the intra-ocular pressure remains under control); severe psychoneuroses or psychoses.

Administration of levodopa with other therapeutic agents

Anticholinergic drugs should be continued during levodopa therapy. As treatment with levodopa proceeds and the therapeutic effect is found, the dosage of the anticholinergic drugs may need to be changed.

Drugs which interfere with central amine mechanisms such as rauwolfia alkaloids (reserpine), phenothiazines, thioxanthenes, butyrophenones, and amphetamines should be avoided where possible. If however, the administration is considered essential, extreme care should be exercised and a close watch kept for any signs of potentiation, antagonism, or other interactions and for any unusual side-effects. It should not be given in conjunction with monoamine oxidase inhibitors, nor within two weeks of their withdrawal. Pyridoxine (vitamin B6), is known to block the effects of levodopa. This is commonly included in multivitamin preparations.

Since the extent of the experience of concomitant levodopa and other drugs is still limited, other interactions may occur. Thus when other drugs must be given in conjunction with levodopa, the patient should be carefully observed for unusual side-effects or potentiating effects. Studies are progressing with the combined administration of levodopa with various inhibitors of peripheral decarboxylase. The clinical data currently available indicates that therapeutic response is attained at a lower dose and possibly with a reduced incidence of side-effects. Levodopa may also be given with amantadine with some benefit; the optimum regimen has still to be determined for each of these combined forms of therapy.

Effects of overdosage and their treatment

Symptoms of overdosage are qualitatively similar to the side-effects but may be of greater magnitude.

Treatment should include gastric lavage, general supportive measures, intravenous fluids and the maintenance of an adequate air way. Electrocardiographic monitoring should be instituted and the patient carefully observed for the possible development of arrhythmias. If necessary, antiarrhythmic therapy should be given, and other symptoms treated as they arise.

Index

Acetylcholine, 100, 146
Adrenaline, 47
    estimation of, 64
Akinesia 59, 62
    paradoxica, 83
    treatment with L-Dopa, 100
Akinetic hypertonic syndrome, 54
Alpha-methyl-dopa (Aldomet), 71, 72, 119
Amantadine, 100, 162
Anticholinergic drugs, 99, 161
    dosage, 110
Anticholinergic withdrawal, 101
    effect on handwriting, 112
    results, 103
Anti-Parkinsonism therapy, 146
Athetoid movements, 91, 95
Atropine, 99
Autonomic 'release' phenomena, 110

Basal ganglia, 2, 63, 132
Benedict's syndrome, 24
Blood-brain barrier, 39, 41, 60, 94, 115
Blood manganese concentrations, 93, 95
Bradykinesia, 106

Catecholamines, 41, 47, 63

daily excretion of, 66
    intracerebral distribution of, 123
    metabolism, 147
urinary estimation of, 65
urinary excretion of, 65, 70
Chemical sympathectomy, 151
Choreoathetoid movements, 83
Cogwheel phenomenon, 88
Corpus striatum, 45, 47, 85, 146

Decarboxylase inhibitors, 115, 118, 125
    chemistry and action of, 119
    effects, 125, 126, 128, 129
Dioxyphenylalanine (DOPA), 31
    d-Dopa, 77
    dl-Dopa, 81, 87
    l-Dopa, 29, 59, 60, 61, 73, 77
    l-Dopa decarboxylase, 147
Dioxyphenylaminopropionic acid, 31, 33
    conversion to protocatechuic acid, 35
    isolation of, 33
    precipitation reactions of, 34, 35
    purification of, 34
    solubility reactions of, 34, 35
Dopa, 54, 86
    effects of, 94

overdosage, 68, 162
Dopa decarboxylase, 70, 115, 119, 147
Dopa therapy, 151
 effect on handwriting, 90
 side effects, 153
Dopacetic acid, 68
Dopamine, 47, 100, 146
 action, 146
 distribution in brain, 49, 54
 levels in brian 45
 levels in corpus striatum, 45
 precursors of, 73, 76
Dopamine-β-hydroxylase, 148
Dopamine-β-oxidase activity, 53
DOPS (*threo*-dihydroxyphenylserine),
 148
Dyskinetic movements, 110

Extrapyramidal disorders, 51, 52
 disease, 85

Gait, 106
 changes in, 108
Granulocytopenia, 81, 96, 152

Homovanillic acid, 63
 secretion, 46
 urinary excretion of, 70
Huntington's chorea, 45, 52, 54, 55
Hypersalivation, 100
Hypokinesia, 82, 153

Iproniazid, 42, 59

Keniadrin, 73

L-Dopa, 73, 87
 effects on rigidity and tremor, 74,
  76, 90, 152
 metabolism of, 68
 toxological effects, 92
L-tyrosine, 29, 147
Lesions,
 arteriosclerotic, 25
 degenerative, 25
 inflammatory, 25
 localisation, of, 22
 nigral, 19, 21

results of, 22
Levodopa (dihydroxy-phenylalanine),
 29, 31, 115
 biochemistry of, 143
 intestinal absorption of, 126, 128
 metabolic pathways for, 4
 metabolism of, 143
 therapeutic effects, 57
Levodopa decarboxylation, 117
Levodopa metabolism
 in animals, 121
 in humans, 127
Levodopa therapy, 102
 dosage, 110, 159
 indications for, 159
 maintenance therapy, 160
 side effects, 82, 153, 160

Lewy bodies, 2, 26
Locus Niger, 21, 22, 27

MAO inhibitors, 59, 71, 73, 149, 161
Melanocyte-stimulating hormone, 85
 action of, 95
 clinical evaluation, 94
 dosages, 86
 laboratory tests, 87
 results of treatment, 88
Melanogenesis, 85
m-hydroxylated amines, 149
Midbrain, 19
Monoamine oxidase, (MAO), 149
Monoplegic paralysis agitans, 27
Motor disorders, 23, 25
Muscular tone disorders, 22, 23

Neostriatum, 53
Noradrenaline, 47
 distribution in brain, 49
 estimation of, 64
 levels in brian, 45, 48

O-methylation, 147
O-methyldopamine, 70
Oral therapy, 81
Orthostatic hypotension, 151

Paralysis agitans, 1, 7

Parkinsonian rigidity, 22
Parkinsonism
    arteriosclerotic, 63, 64
    causes, 2, 145
    characteristics, 1, 7, 145
    clinical features, 2
    iatrogenic, 1
    idiopathic, 19, 45, 64, 102, 152
    pathogenesis of, 21
    postencephalitic, 45, 50, 63, 64,
      152, 160
    unilateral, 19, 25

Parnate, 73
    effects of, 70, 74
Pyridoxine (Vitamin B6), 161

Reserpine, 39, 41, 59, 72, 146, 161
Rigidity, 106
    evaluation of, 64
RO4-4602, 115
RO4-4602-levodopa therapy, 133
    biochemical side effects, 139
    clinical side effects, 138
    methods, 134
    results, 136

Serotonin (5-HT), 41, 47, 59, 117, 151
    metabolism of, 128
Shaking palsy, 1, 7, 9
    causes of, 15
    history of, 11
    pathognomonic symptoms, 14
    treatment, 16
Stereotactic surgery, 99
Substantia nigra, 2, 19, 85, 146
Sympathin, 47

Threo-dihydroxyphenylserine (DOPS),
    148
Tremor, 106
    evaluation of, 64
Tremor tenulentus, 15
Tyrosine, 73

Urinary volume, 66

Vanillin, 29
Vacuolisation, of bone marrow cells, 86,
    96
Vicia faba, 31
Vitanun B6, 70

Wilson's disease, 24